THE
Chemotherapy
SURVIVAL GUIDE

JUDITH McKAY, R.N.
NANCEE HIRANO, R.N., M.S.N.

NEW HARBINGER PUBLICATIONS, INC.

Publisher's Note

This publication is designed to provide accurate and authoritative information in regard to the subject matter covered. It is sold with the understanding that the publisher is not engaged in rendering psychological, financial, legal, or other professional services. If expert assistance or counseling is needed, the services of a competent professional should be sought.

Drawings on pages 46, 47, 52, and 53 used with the permission of Abbott Laboratories and originally appeared in their booklet "Venous Access Device Occlusions." Drawings on pages 49 and 51 adapted from "Venous Access Device Occlusions" by SHELBY DESIGNS & ILLUSTRATES.

Library of Congress Catalog Number: 93-084710
ISBN 1-879237-57-1 Paperback
ISBN 1-879237-58-x Hardcover

Copyright © by New Harbinger Publications, Inc.
            5674 Shattuck Avenue
            Oakland, CA 94609

Printed in the United States of America on recycled paper.

Edited by Kirk Johnson
Cover design by SHELBY DESIGNS & ILLUSTRATES

First printing September, 1993, 5,000 copies
Second printing November, 1993, 5,000 copies
Third printing February, 1994, 5,000 copies

For my husband Matthew,
      and to the memory of my father, Benjamin Becker.

—J. Mc.

For my husband, Terence Shinsato, to the memory of my mother-in-law, Grace Shinsato, and for Buffy.

—N.H.

Acknowledgments

We are grateful to the following people who've been extremely helpful in the development of this book. Kirk Johnson for his fine editing, Dr. Janet Lyle, Clinical Oncology Pharmacist, who reviewed several chapters for accuracy and clarity, Dr. Michael Cassidy, Dr. Gary Cecchi and Holly Schenck, R.N. for valuable feedback, Mary Hoffman for her contributions to the stress reduction chapter, Eli Leon for his editorial assistance, and Marcy McGaugh for word processing. We are especially appreciative to Dr. Matthew McKay who helped at every stage of writing and editing.

We would also like to thank our patients who, by sharing their experiences with us, gave us a better understanding of how we could help others.

Contents

Introduction

A survival guide is a book of directions to help travelers cope with difficulties or unusual circumstances. It provides essential information, practical suggestions, and encouragement so that travelers can use their own resources and the resources in their environment to make it through the obstacles along the way.

Many people who are facing chemotherapy for the first time feel like they have been dropped behind enemy lines during a war. They don't know the language or the terrain and don't know what to expect or what is expected of them. The hospital or clinic environment and technical medical terminology are foreign. All of these circumstances add to the feeling of being lost in an alien world. A person recovering from the stress of recent cancer surgery may feel even more overwhelmed. And it may be difficult to get needed support if friends and family are busy dealing with their own fears and misconceptions about cancer and chemotherapy.

This book is meant to be a survival guide. It explains what chemotherapy is, how it works, and how it may affect you. It contains simple and understandable answers for many of the questions you may have. Most importantly, it gives you practical suggestions about what you can do to help yourself while receiving chemotherapy. These are the same hints and suggestions that nurses give their patients based on their experience and the experiences of the many people who have gone through these treatments.

Before the Era of Chemotherapy

Chemotherapy is the term used to identify the various drugs that fight cancer. It is a relatively new science, with pioneering treatments beginning in the early 1950s. Before chemotherapy, the most common treatment for cancer was surgery. But if the cancer was in an area that couldn't be surgically removed, or if some cancer cells had spread to other areas of the body, no effective treatment was available. In those days, surgery tended to be more "radical," often removing large areas of healthy tissue in an attempt to catch the few microscopic cancer cells that might have escaped the original tumor.

How Chemotherapy Began

One distinguishing characteristic of most cancer cells is their tendency to divide frequently—too frequently, in a way that is out of control. This tendency means that any drug that can damage cells in the dividing stage will have a far greater effect on cancer cells than most normal tissue. The first chemical therapy treatments used this principle to kill quickly dividing cancer cells in the blood (leukemia) and the lymph system (lymphoma). Since then, more than fifty cancer-fighting drugs have been developed based on this same approach. Researchers continue to explore how these drugs can be used alone and in combination with other drugs to make this form of treatment even more successful.

Current Uses of Chemotherapy

Modern chemotherapy is a powerful and in many cases highly effective weapon in the fight against cancer. It has become a major component of the first line of attack to prevent the spread of the disease and can significantly improve the chances for recovery. For some kinds of cancer that are particularly vulnerable to the effects of chemotherapy, it may be the *only* treatment necessary. To increase its effectiveness, many people also receive chemotherapy in conjunction with other forms of treatment such as surgery, radiation, or hormonal therapy. Chemotherapy is often used even when all measurable signs of cancer are gone. This is just to make sure that any possible spread of cancer cells—even on a microscopic level—is eliminated.

What This Book Offers

Most people know very little about what to expect when they are getting chemotherapy. They may be aware of some potential side effects such as nausea or hair loss, but they don't know whether these reactions will happen to them or what if anything they can do about them.

The purpose of this book is to answer many of your questions about chemotherapy. Moreover, it offers guidance for how you can help yourself during your treatment. What does chemotherapy feel like? How is it given? What should you do before, during, and after each treatment? What can you expect at home? Why do you need so many blood tests? And what do the tests show about how your body is reacting to the chemotherapy?

You do not need to read this book from beginning to end, but, you can turn to any chapter for information and suggestions about the specific issue that concerns you.

At the heart of the guide are chapters describing the different side effects that might occur because of chemotherapy's impact on healthy cells. At the beginning of each of these chapters is a review of how chemotherapy works and why it can cause that specific side effect. These sections are followed by many suggestions of what you can do to prevent, minimize, or manage the side effect. Accompanying these coping chapters is a chapter focusing on how to maintain good nutrition even when you are experiencing temporary changes in your appetite or digestion.

No traveler is ever entirely alone, and Chapter 10 contains some crucial ideas for getting support from your family and friends as well as descriptions of several kinds of support groups that you may want to consider joining. Chapter 11 explains how you can use relaxation and stress reduction techniques to lower your anxiety, and Chapter 12 contains a script you can use to make your own audiotape for healing visualizations.

What This Book Can't Do

Your doctor will prescribe specific chemotherapy medications and dosages based on the kind of cancer you have, its location, and its cellular characteristics, as well as your age, physical condition, and how well you are tolerating the treatment. Because there are so many different drugs, dosages, and combinations that are now used to fight cancer, this book doesn't include descriptions of each drug. Your doctor or nurse will provide you with that specific information and review the potential side effects with you.

This book is not a substitute for calling the doctor if you have a problem. There are many things about your specific treatment or symptoms that may need your immediate attention. What you may consider to be "just a little cough and a cold" may require antibiotics or lab tests when you are taking chemo-therapy. An ache or swelling or rash can also be more significant during chemotherapy. So don't be shy about calling with a problem or symptom or question. Keep in mind that you will probably develop a closer connection with your oncologist (the specialist in cancer care) than you have had with other physicians in the past.

Chemotherapy treatments are stressful, both physically and emotionally. But if you know what to expect, you will feel less overwhelmed. If you understand what problems may arise and what you can do to feel better, you will feel more empowered. If you are armed with practical suggestions and a coping plan to deal with problems, you can feel more in control. This survival guide can help make the journey easier by providing the information and sources of support you need to face the challenge and make it through.

1

What Is Chemotherapy?

In order to understand how chemotherapy will help you, you first must understand how cancer cells are different from normal cells. You need to understand how cancer cells grow and how their growth can be stopped.

A Primer on Cell Life

All living things are made up of cells, and each cell has a life of its own. Cells are the basic building blocks of life. When you look at a one-cell organism (like the amoeba you saw under the microscope in biology class), you can identify different cell structures that keep the cell working, dividing, and surviving. A *cell wall* surrounds the cell and separates it from its environment and determines what goes in and what goes out. Within the cell is a very important structure called the *nucleus*, the cell's command center. The nucleus directs and controls all of a cell's functions and determines how and when it divides. Within the nucleus is the DNA, which is like a master computer program for that cell.

When the cell divides, it splits into two identical pieces. First, the DNA splits in half and duplicates itself, so that each half will have a complete and identical DNA program for that cell. Then the cell membrane and all the other structures divide. Each new daughter cell is exactly like the original parent cell, with identical cell parts, nucleus, and DNA information.

Complex life forms like ourselves are made up of millions of cells. Groups of cells perform different specialized functions to keep the whole system working well. Some are part of the heart muscle and have the ability to contract. Other cells are part of the digestive system and secrete enzymes or absorb nutrients. Some are part of the liver and function to filter the blood and store energy. But all cells work together to keep the big system, the human body, alive and well in its environment. All cells are living, growing, and at times dividing in a specific and controlled way based on a program contained in the DNA.

Characteristics of Normal Cells

Normal cells grow in a limited space and stay within their boundaries. Bone cells don't grow into the muscles that surround them; stomach cells don't grow into the space that the pancreas occupies (even though they lie right next to each other).

Normal cells divide at a set and controlled rate, depending on their function, their life span, and the information contained in their DNA. Some cells have a short life span and divide frequently. For example, the life span for some white blood cells is only 72 hours. The life span for a cell in your intestines is only 2 weeks. Other cells have a longer life span. The average red blood cell will live 3 months.

Some cells live as long as you do, dividing only to replace themselves if there has been an injury. For instance, if an adult breaks his arm, the bone cells are "turned on" to repair the damage. Once the injury heals, then bone cells in an adult divide very rarely. In fact, there are some cells which never divide again once they have grown to adult size. Brain cells do not divide and replace themselves even when damaged. The rate that normal cells divide is specific to each group and strictly controlled by their DNA program. This program is different for each type of cell.

Normal cells have a tendency to stick together so that cells do not break off and float away even though the blood flows by each and every cell. If a normal cell were to break off into the blood and lodge elsewhere in the body, it would soon die. Normal cells are "well differentiated," meaning that a pathologist can easily identify what kind of cell it is, what it does, and where it comes from. Liver cells look different than bladder cells; bone cells are quite distinct from brain cells. Cells with different functions vary as to size, shape, and diameter of the nucleus.

How Cells Are Nourished

Every one of the body's cells is washed continuously with blood. The blood carries oxygen from the lungs and nutrients from the digestive system. The blood is pumped by the heart through big arteries, then smaller and smaller vessels, until the blood reaches each and every cell, delivering oxygen and energy. Then, the blood picks up waste products which are produced by the cells and carries them to the filtering and cleansing organs (kidney, liver, lung) to be recycled or eliminated by the body. Every time you exhale, you get rid of some of the waste products (carbon dioxide) of cell activity. And when you urinate, you are eliminating waste products filtered out by your kidneys. Your blood is really a kind of transport system that trucks in life-sustaining supplies and then hauls off the debris.

How Cells Are Protected

The immune system provides mobile defenses for the body, sending out white blood cells (soldier cells) that seek and destroy bacteria and viruses. White blood cells are mixed in the blood and wash along with it past every cell. They gather at the site of infections, surrounding and killing bacteria and viruses, and eventually migrate by way of lymph ducts to the lymph glands (or lymph nodes).

Lymph nodes are like a cluster of grapes, and act as filtering stations at various locations in your body. Each cluster of nodes receives lymphocytes that have washed past a certain organ. The nodes are the places where the bacteria, worn-out lymphocytes, and debris are filtered and destroyed. You aren't usually aware of your lymph nodes unless they are swollen and tender from fighting infection. For example, you might feel swollen lymph nodes in your neck or under your jaw from a sore throat or an infected tooth. You might feel lymph nodes in your groin from a pelvic infection or in your armpit from an infection in your hand. Doctors know where to find the particular cluster of lymph nodes that filter each organ. They know where to feel for signs of infection and which lymph nodes to examine under the microscope when looking for cancer cells.

Characteristics of Cancer Cells

Cancer begins as a mutation or change in the DNA of a single normal cell in any part of the body. Once this change takes place, the set of instructions in the DNA is changed and the cell no longer acts like it normally does. Often a mutation or change results in a cell so damaged that it cannot survive or it fails to divide successfully. But if it does survive and divide, that mutated cell may look and act very differently from the cells around it.

Cancer cells look different. They may have a different size or shape or have larger or smaller nuclei. They may not fit together in an orderly, predictable arrangement of cells. They may not be able to do the job that they were designed to do.

Cancer cells often ignore the normal rate of cell division because they lack a growth control mechanism. They may divide very rapidly, crowding, pushing, or blocking other organs and preventing them from doing their job. Because they don't stay within their boundaries, but instead, grow into surrounding organs, they are said to be *invasive*. Cancer cells frequently appear immature because they may divide several times before they are fully grown. They are also more likely to mutate again.

Whereas normal cells have a tendency to stick together, cancer cells are more likely to detach from the original location and move via the bloodstream to other areas of the body. They are also more likely to travel by way of the lymph system to the lymph nodes downstream and then to other organ systems. Most of these detached cells are usually destroyed by the body's defense system or filtered and eliminated like bacteria and other cell debris. But if the detached cancer cells do survive, they may produce a new growth at a different site or damage other organs as well.

Some Terms You Should Know

Hyperplasia is an increase in the number of cells at a particular site. It's a normal response to healing a broken bone or a surgical scar. It means that the cells are growing and dividing more quickly until the bone or scar is healed, when growth can slow down to its usual pace. The cells grow in an orderly, regular way and are easily identifiable (well differentiated). They look and act like normal cells.

Dysplasia is an overgrowth of cells that do not have the normal arrangement or function of normal cells. *Neoplasia* means new growth and describes the growth of cells beyond their normal boundaries. These new cells may be cancerous (malignant) or noncancerous (benign). Noncancerous overgrowth is well differentiated, and the cells look similar to other normal cells of the same organ. Such a growth usually divides slowly and is often encased in a limited area. It doesn't invade the tissue around it, nor will it travel to any other parts of the body. A benign cyst is an example of a noncancerous neoplasia.

A malignant tumor is an overgrowth of cells that often looks very dissimilar to normal cells in that organ. The cells may appear immature, divide quickly, and grow in a less orderly way. They may not be enclosed in a limited area and can invade the surrounding tissue. They can also detach from the tumor into the lymph system or the blood system and migrate to distant parts of the body. Some may survive and begin dividing in this new region.

When a little bit of tumor is removed and examined under a microscope, this procedure is called a *biopsy*. A pathologist will look at a few cells from the tumor to see how they compare to normal cells of that organ. He can determine whether the tumor has invaded surrounding tissue. By looking at nearby lymph glands, he can see if parts of the tumor have detached and are growing there.

Cancerous cells that have detached and traveled by the blood or lymph system usually cannot survive the blood pressure or the body's defense systems. Occasionally, however, they may lodge in an area where the blood pressure is low and blood moves slowly. The cancerous cells may grow there. This spread of cancer cells to another distant organ site is called *metastasis*.

From the very beginning, the doctor wants to know everything he can about the cancer. He gets that information with the help of many tests, including a biopsy, X-rays, scans, and blood tests. Sometimes even the DNA of the cancerous cell is examined. This information-gathering process is called *staging*. The results of all the tests will determine what kind of treatment you need.

Some cancerous cells produce substances that can be measured by a simple blood test. These substances are called *tumor markers* because they indicate the presence of cancer cells, even if the cells cannot be seen. If a tumor marker measures higher than normal, it indicates an increase in cancer cells. When the tumor marker drops lower, it usually indicates that there are fewer of these cells and that the tumor is "responding" to treatment. The doctor uses the tumor marker as important data in treatment decisions.

Treatment

Surgery. This is the oldest method of treating cancer, and sometimes it is the only treatment necessary. This is more likely to be true if the cancer is small, contained, and has not spread to adjacent tissue or spread through the lymph system or the blood system. At the time of surgery, the tumor is removed along with some of the healthy surrounding tissue. Often lymph nodes from adjacent areas are also removed so that the pathologist can see if they have some cancerous cells growing in them.

If the cancer has spread, or if it is an aggressive type of cancer with a high likelihood of spreading to other organs, additional anticancer treatments may be recommended. In many cases, these additional treatments are recommended even if the original cancer is small, contained, and shows no sign of spreading to other areas.

Radiation. This treatment uses high energy particles that can penetrate through your body. Special machines generate and direct these particles to a specific place for a specific amount of time. Radiation therapy uses high energy particles similar to X-rays which, in tiny doses, create chest or dental films for diagnostic purposes.

A specialist (the radiation oncologist) calculates the exact area, amount, and frequency of radiation treatments based on the kind of tumor, location, biopsies, and so on. Normal tissues are shielded, and the radiation beam is precisely aimed at the tumor so it gets a high dose of radiation and the normal tissue does not. Cells that are dividing quickly, like cancer cells, are especially sensitive to radiation. When these high energy particles are directed at a tumor site, they damage or destroy these cells. Radiation damages the cell's DNA, cell membranes, and other cell structures.

Radiation may be the only treatment necessary if the cancer cells are very sensitive to its effects and there is no sign that the cancer has spread. Radiation treatment may also be given before surgery to shrink a tumor so it can more easily be removed. Or, it may be given along with or following chemotherapy because some of the chemotherapy medicines make cancer cells more sensitive to the effects of radiation. Radiation may be suggested after surgery even if there are no detectable cancer cells in the lymph or surrounding tissue just to make sure no cells have escaped.

Chemotherapy. The medicines used to treat cancer include a large group of different drugs. Some—like hormones and steroids—have familiar uses other than the treatment of cancer. But any drug or combination of drugs that kills, slows down, or damages cancer cells can be considered chemotherapy.

You are familiar with medicines that treat bacterial infection, such as antibiotics. Once they enter your bloodstream, these drugs have little effect on the rest of your body. It is the bacteria that are sensitive to and are killed by the antibiotics. But since cancer cells are not a foreign invader, but, instead are damaged, mutated human cells, anticancer medicine has to work in a different way. It has to kill cancer cells *without permanently damaging* normal cells.

No current anticancer medicine attacks just cancer cells without affecting some normal cells. The cells affected have the same characteristic that makes cancer cells vulnerable to radiation. Since chemotherapy damages cancer cells that are rapidly dividing, those normal cells that are dividing rapidly are also affected by the drugs.

Some chemotherapy drugs interfere with the sequence of activities that a cell must go through to divide into two identical daughter cells. If the cell can't divide, then it will live out its life span and die. Drugs that act this way are called *cell cycle specific*. They prevent cancer cells from reproducing at a particular phase of the cell's life span.

Other chemotherapy drugs affect cancer cells in all phases of life. But because cancer cells are often more immature or fragile than normal cells, these drugs affect cancer cells far more than healthy cells. These medicines are called *cell cycle nonspecific* since they kill cancer cells at any time during their life span without waiting for them to divide. These drugs are especially useful in killing cancer cells that are slow growing.

Other drugs can make the environment less hospitable to cancer cells and thus slow them down. Hormones work this way. For instance, some breast cancer tumors grow faster in the presence of estrogen, and some prostate cancer grows faster in the presence of testosterone. Hormones that block estrogen or testosterone can discourage the growth of the cancer cells.

Combinations of drugs.   Years ago people were usually given one chemotherapy drug at a time. Now, with further research and the development of new drugs, doctors may recommend a combination of chemotherapy drugs. This combination of drugs can often be more effective at killing cancer cells than using one drug alone. Anticancer drugs with different modes of action and which produce different side effects are usually combined. For instance, you may be given a chemotherapy drug that kills the cancer cells while they are dividing. You may also be given a chemotherapy drug which kills cells even when they are not dividing. You may also take a hormone which will change the environment of the cancer cells and discourage their growth.

Using a combination of drugs that work in different ways can make chemotherapy *more deadly* to cancer cells and *less toxic* to healthy cells. The combination of drugs and the schedule of how frequently you get treatments depends on the kind of cancer, its location, and how quickly your healthy cells recover from the treatment.

Side Effects

You take medicine for some desired effect. Different medicines can lower blood pressure, relieve pain, kill bacteria, and so on. The effects are usually predictable and beneficial. But medicines often have other effects which may be predictable, but are not necessarily beneficial. Side effects are undesired consequences that inevitably occur when taking certain medicines.

For instance, while the predictable and beneficial effect of a narcotic is to relieve pain, one of its side effects is sleepiness. You are often informed of the side effects of common medications when they are prescribed.

As you are aware, chemotherapy works by damaging cells that are dividing frequently. But other noncancerous cell populations in the body are also dividing frequently. These are cells of the bone marrow (where blood cells are made) and the mucous membranes of the gastrointestinal (GI) tract (from the mouth to the large intestines). Hair follicles also divide quickly and are sensitive to some chemotherapy medicines. The side effects of chemotherapy reflect the effect that anticancer medicine has on *all* fast-growing cell populations. Most chemotherapy medicine temporarily affects the ability of the bone marrow to produce blood cells, including the white blood cells that fight infection. Some chemotherapy medicines temporarily cause gastrointestinal disturbances such as diarrhea or nausea and vomiting. Some chemotherapy medicines cause temporary hair loss or hair thinning.

The kind of side effects you may experience depends on the kind of chemotherapy drugs you are getting, the dose, and the frequency of your treatments. Your doctor and nurse will tell you what you can expect. It is most important to remember that chemotherapy's side effects, the disruption to healthy cells, is time limited and temporary. Some side effects are preventable. For instance, the side effect of nausea can often be prevented by taking antinausea medication before you start taking an anticancer drug and for several doses afterwards. Some side effects cannot be prevented, but there are many things that you can do to minimize, treat, or manage the side effects. Preventing and managing the side effects of chemotherapy is a very important part of your treatment plan and will help you live a normal, active life. Your GI system, hair, and blood-manufacturing capabilities will return to normal after your treatment is over.

Chapters 4 to 9 will tell you much more about the possible side effects of chemotherapy and how to cope with them. They explain why the side effects occur, and how to prevent, relieve, or manage the problems if they develop.

2

Understanding
Blood Tests

When you are ill, it seems that everyone is after your blood. Every time you look up there's someone in a lab coat, carrying a tourniquet and multicolored test tubes, who needs just a few more ounces. You wonder why so many tests? Why so often? You may even feel that you are giving too much blood and worry how and when your body will replace it.

You have about four to five quarts of blood in your body, and most blood tests require only about a teaspoon of blood in each test tube. The few teaspoons of blood you lose each time blood is drawn for a test are rapidly replaced. Even someone donating a pint of blood replaces it so quickly that he or she can donate again in about two weeks.

This chapter covers some of the most frequent blood tests that your doctor may order. Many of them can be done at the same time, with only one needle stick. The nurse or lab technicians can simply keep the needle in place and change the collection tubes. Then the samples can be sent to different departments in the lab for analysis. Unfortunately, there are times, especially when you are a patient in the hospital, that no sooner does the lab technician leave, than another comes in for another test and another needle stick! But as a rule, your doctors and nurses try to consolidate the tests so that doesn't happen.

In the hospital, routine blood tests are usually drawn very early in the morning around 6 a.m. This is a source of great annoyance to many people, since they can't imagine why samples must be taken at such an ungodly hour. The reason blood samples are collected so early is that it takes several hours for the lab to perform all the tests and get the results to the nurse's station and into your chart. When the doctors come each day to review your chart and determine what medications, IVs, treatments, or tests you need, the results of blood tests are an important source of information.

Don't hesitate to ask your nurse or doctor what blood tests are being done and why they are necessary. You also may want to know the results of the tests and what they indicate about your condition. Some people even keep notes about their blood tests—which tests were done, why they were done, and the results.

Why Test Your Blood?

Blood is the fluid of life. It carries oxygen from your lungs to each and every cell of your body. It carries the glucose that all your cells need for energy and then carries off the waste products from the cells' activities. Blood contains your body's defense against infection and carries the means of repairing the vessels (arteries and veins) in which it flows. Blood maintains the balance of all the chemicals that are necessary for muscles and nerves to function and provides the communication and co-ordination for all your organs to work together. With these diverse functions, you can see why a small sample of your blood provides an amazing window into the health and functioning of every organ within you. A mere teaspoon or two, when analyzed by the lab, can tell a great deal about you.

Blood is made of cells and plasma. The blood cells are red cells, white cells, and platelets, which are all produced in your bone marrow. The plasma is a straw-colored fluid containing blood cells along with chemicals, enzymes, minerals, vitamins, hormones, and everything else your body needs to stay alive. A *complete blood count* (CBC) identifies the types, quantities, and characteristics of the different cells of your blood. A *blood chemistry* analyzes the plasma.

Bone Marrow—The Blood Cell Factory

Bone marrow is the tissue within your bones where blood cells are made. In infants, all the bone marrow is capable of manufacturing blood cells. But in adults, blood cells are made only in the flat bones of the pelvis, sternum (breast bone), and skull.

The bone marrow is like a blood cell factory. It contains *stem cells* that have the capacity to evolve into all three types of blood cells. A stem cell can develop into a red cell and carry oxygen. Or it can evolve into a white cell and fight infection. Or it can evolve into a platelet, which can stop bleeding by forming a clot.

Bone marrow maintains the normal number of the three types of cells by replacing old cells as they naturally die off and increasing production of any kind of blood cell if there is a special demand for it. For instance, your bone marrow will step up production of white cells when you have an infection.

The bone marrow is a place where cells are dividing very quickly in order to keep up with your body's constant demand for blood cells of all kinds. Since chemotherapy affects the cells that are dividing quickly (like cancer cells), it will temporarily affect your bone marrow. Unlike cancer cells, your bone marrow will recover and resume its normal production of blood cells.

Chemotherapy doesn't affect the blood cells that are already in circulation, since they are not dividing. Only the production of new cells in the bone marrow is slowed down. Chemotherapy's effect on your bone marrow usually shows up in your blood cell count about a week to ten days after your treatment. That is when you can see that the blood cells have not been replaced at the normal rate. But in another week or so, the number of blood cells in circulation will return to normal.

Your chemotherapy treatments are timed to allow your bone marrow to recover. Your doctor will always check your blood cell count before each treatment to be sure that your bone marrow is back on the job of producing blood cells.

Red Cells

Your red cells (also called erythrocytes) give blood its color. Ninety percent of each red cell is made up of hemoglobin, a substance rich in iron. The size, shape, and flexibility of red cells enable them to squeeze through the small openings between cells. The red cells' purpose is to carry oxygen from your lungs to every corner of your body. If you have too few red cells because of blood loss or because your bone marrow is not working normally, then your body's ability to carry oxygen is jeopardized.

When your red blood cell count is low, your heart has to work harder to cycle the remaining red cells at a faster rate to provide your body with the oxygen it needs. You may feel tired, since there may not be enough oxygen to keep up with the activity of your muscles. You may feel dizzy when you stand up after you have been sitting or lying down. You may chill easier or feel winded more easily after exerting yourself. These are all symptoms that your body needs more oxygen and more red cells to carry it.

Red cells have a relatively long life span (about three or four months). While the production of new red cells is slowed down for a few days after your chemotherapy, the fact that red cells live so long makes the problem much less severe. By the time more cells are needed, your bone marrow has long since recovered and has usually caught up.

A complete blood count (CBC) provides three measurements that reflect the adequacy of your red cells. They are the red blood cell count (RBC), hemoglobin (HGB), and hematocrit (HCT).

The red blood cell count is the number of red cells in a cubic millimeter of blood. The normal amount of red cells is about 4.5 to 6 million per cubic millimeter for men and 4 to 5.5 million per cubic millimeter for women. The normal values for women are less than for men because women who are menstruating lose a small amount of blood each month with their periods.

The hemoglobin (HGB) test measures the amount of this substance in a sample of blood. Hemoglobin is the part of a red cell that actually carries the oxygen, so an HGB test gives a good indication of the red cells' ability to carry oxygen from the lungs to all the parts of your body. Normal hemoglobin for men is from 14 to 18 grams per 100 milligrams of blood. For women it is slightly less (12 to 16 grams).

The hematocrit (HCT) measurement determines what percent of the sample of whole blood contains red cells. Normally red cells comprise 42 to 54 percent for men and 38 to 46 percent for women.

If you have lost a lot of blood or your red blood production has been slowed down, then all three tests will be lower than normal. As your body turns up the production of red cells in the bone marrow or you receive a blood transfusion of red cells, all three values will rise.

What To Do When Your Red Cell Count Is Low

Many people get through chemotherapy without having a noticeable drop in the production of their red cells. Since the red cells live for so long and the bone marrow recovers in four to ten days, they are soon replaced. Depending on your general health, you may be able to cope with a mild drop in red cells without noticing anything more than fatigue.

If your red cells do get low, you'll need to rest more and eat well—especially foods high in iron. Your doctor may prescribe an iron supplement. If you don't have enough cells to carry normal amounts of oxygen to your brain, you may feel dizzy for a few minutes when first standing up from a lying position. If that happens, you should get up slowly and take some deep breaths until the dizziness subsides.

Stimulating Red Blood Cell Production

A special hormone stimulates bone marrow to produce red cells. This hormone, erythropoietin, is normally produced by the kidneys in response to a drop in the oxygen carrying capacity of the blood. Erythropoietin works by stimulating the red blood cells to mature faster. A synthetic version of this hormone can be given by injection to speed up red cell production when it has been slowed by the effects of chemotherapy. If you have a severe drop in your red cells, you may require a blood transfusion.

White Cells

White blood cells (leukocytes) provide your body's defense from infection. White cells are produced and stored in the bone marrow and are released when the body needs them. Once in the bloodstream, they circulate for only about twelve hours. Any inflammation or bacterial invasion will attract these cells, triggering them to leave the bloodstream and gather at the site of infection. There they surround the bacteria or other foreign body like an amoeba, stretching and wrapping themselves around it and then digesting it. White cells also help damaged tissue repair itself.

There are five kinds of white cells that are produced in the bone marrow. The first three (neutrophils, eosinophils, and basophils) have a granular appearance when seen under a microscope, and because of that they are called granulocytes. The two other types of white cells are lymphocytes and monocytes.

Neutrophils.   Neutrophils are the most numerous white blood cells. They comprise 62 percent of all white cells and are the first to gather at an infection. Their job is to localize and neutralize bacteria. Each neutrophil can inactivate from five to twenty bacteria. When neutrophils are used up from fighting bacteria they rupture, and the contents of the ruptured cell attracts even more neutrophils, as well as increasing the blood supply to that area. The increased blood circulation can make an infected area appear redder and feel hotter than usual.

Eosinophils.   Eosinophils are the white cells that respond to allergic reactions. Their job is to detoxify foreign proteins before they can harm the body. They also contain toxic granules that can kill invading cells and clean up areas of inflammation.

Basophils.   Basophils, the rarest of the white cells, release histamine, which increases blood supply and attracts other white cells to the infected area. Basophils make it easier for white cells to migrate out of the blood into the damaged area. They also release heparin, which dissolves old clots.

Lymphocytes.   Lymphocytes not only fight infection, but also provide you with immunity to certain diseases. For example, the measles virus is an antigen—a substance that your body recognizes as foreign. Lymphocytes react to that foreign substance by forming antibodies. Antibodies are proteins which are designed to kill one specific antigen. There are many kinds of antigens, and your lymphocytes develop many different kinds of antibodies to attack them. These antibodies not only fight the foreign substance, but *remember* it so they can kill it whenever you are exposed to it again. Even if it is many years after your first exposure, the antibodies made by your lymphocytes remember the antigen and provide immunity.

Lymphocytes can be produced by the bone marrow or by other organs, such as the lymph glands, spleen, tonsils, or the thymus gland. They move back and forth between your blood and your lymph system. While many lymphocytes produce antibodies, others function as regulators for your immune response—either helping it or suppressing it, depending on how well you are fighting an infection.

Monocytes. The last type of white blood cells are the body's second line of defense because they do not respond as quickly as neutrophils. Their job is to move into an infected area to remove damaged or dying cells or cell debris. They contain special enzymes that are very effective in killing bacteria. Monocytes are produced in the bone marrow and initially circulate in your blood. Once they leave the blood, they go into the tissue and establish themselves in the lymph nodes, lungs, liver, or spleen.

Signs of Infection

All five kinds of white cells work together to fight infection. The usual signs of infection are swelling, redness, and warmth in the affected area and fever. These symptoms indicate that your immune system is working, fighting bacteria or other foreign organisms. The formation of pus in an infection is really a collection of old, dead bacteria and exhausted white cell debris.

Unlike red cells, which live for months, white cells have a life span of only three or four days, and the bone marrow is constantly producing new cells to replace them. It is the bone marrow's production of white cells that is most vulnerable to the effects of chemotherapy. White cells that are already in circulation or in your tissues are not affected because they are not dividing. But when these cells die off and the reserves have been used up (within one week after your chemotherapy), your white count reaches its lowest point. This period, which is called the *nadir*, occurs about a week to ten days after you get your chemotherapy depending on what kind of chemotherapy you received. It is the time when you are most susceptible to infection. If you are exposed to bacteria during that time, your immune system may not be able to make as strong a response because there are just fewer white cells to respond. Following the nadir, your bone marrow will begin to catch up with white cell production and your count will recover. Your white count returns to normal about three weeks after your chemotherapy.

Your doctor expects your white count to drop temporarily and to recover before your next treatment. But he or she will always check your white count before you get chemotherapy again. If there is a delay in your white cells' recovery, your doctor will delay your treatment for a few days and then check your count again. After several chemotherapy treatments it is not unusual for your white count to be a little sluggish in returning to normal.

What To Do When Your White Count Is Low

Many people who are getting chemotherapy weather the period of time when their white cell counts are low without problem. But you do need to take special precautions to avoid infection during this time. Here's what to do:

- Stay away from anyone who has a cold, flu, or other infection. Stay away from large crowds of people in an enclosed environment to avoid being exposed to coughs and sneezes.

- Keep your skin clean and dry. Moisture provides a breeding place for bacteria. You carry many germs on your hands, so be sure to wash your hands often, especially after using the toilet. Remind others (doctors, nurses, or anyone else helping with your care) to wash their hands too. Keep your teeth and gums clean as well. The food left on your teeth or under your dentures is a place bacteria could grow.

- Drink plenty of fluids, since urinating frequently will keep your bladder from developing an infection.

- Take special care to wash and disinfect any break in your skin and let your doctor know about all but the most superficial cuts. Since it is the action of your white cells that causes inflammation, redness, or pus, you may *not* have these familiar signs of infections while your white cell count is low. You may have an infection and not even know it.

- Check with your doctor if you have any signs of a cold, cough, flu, or fever during this time as well. He or she may want you to take an antibiotic to help your body fight infection more effectively.

When all your chemotherapy treatments are over, your body's defenses will return to normal. But during this time, any exposure or risk of infections should be treated aggressively.

Stimulating White Blood Cell Production

Special proteins in your body called colony stimulating factor (CSF) stimulate the production of white cells. New techniques in genetic engineering have produced different forms of this protein that can be given by injection to counteract the effects of chemotherapy on the body's immune system. There are several forms of CSF that increase different white cells such as granulocytes (G-CSF) and macrophages (M-CSF). When this stimulating factor is given, it causes your bone marrow to speed up the maturation of white cells and shortens the period of time when you are vulnerable to infection.

Not everyone getting chemotherapy will need this medicine to stimulate white blood cell production. But if there is a delay in bone marrow recovery or a high risk of infection, CSF can help your bone marrow recover sooner.

Infections

You are surrounded by a world you cannot see. All around you are bacteria, molds, yeasts, and viruses that can only be observed under a microscope. Everything you touch or eat and even the lining of your digestive system is teeming with microorganisms that could cause infection if they were to penetrate into your blood or tissues.

It is your intact skin and mucous membranes that usually keep these microorganisms from invading your blood system. It is only when these natural barriers are compromised that you risk infection. Your immune system then becomes your next line of defense, mobilizing to fight infection that has penetrated your skin or mucous membranes.

If an infection is severe or your immune system is compromised, you may need some help to fight it. Antibiotics are medicines that help your body fight bacteria infections. There are a number of different antibiotics, and some are more effective in killing certain bacteria than others. Your doctor may want to determine the exact bacteria that is causing your infection so he can prescribe the best antibiotic. He does this by ordering a *culture*.

Getting a Culture

You are probably familiar with throat cultures to determine what kind of organism is causing a sore throat. The doctor or nurse will take a sterile swab and wipe the back of your throat with it. Then the swab is smeared across a nutrient-rich gel and placed in a warm environment to encourage the bacteria to grow rapidly. In a day or two there are enough bacteria growing in the nutrient so that they can be examined under a microscope.

The microbiologist in the lab can then see the exact bacteria causing the problem and determine which antibiotic will be most effective in killing it. When this test is done, it is called a *culture* (the process of growing the bacteria in a nutrient) and *sensitivity* (the process of determining which antibiotics are most effective in killing that bacteria). Viruses, molds, and yeasts can be cultured as well.

Bacteria and other organisms can be cultured from anything your body produces, such as urine, sputum, stool, or drainage from wounds. Blood cultures are quite common. If you have a fever or any other sign of infection, your doctor may want to determine if bacteria (or other organisms) are present in your blood. A sample of your blood is taken and put in an environment which encourages microorganisms to grow. Since your blood supply is so large, it's often difficult to capture a particular organism in a small sample. Accordingly, you may have to have two samples of blood taken a few minutes apart to improve the chances of finding something.

If your infection is severe or your level of infection-fighting white cells is low, your doctor may not wait until the exact bacteria has been identified. After a sample of blood has been taken, he or she may want you to start taking an antibiotic right away. Usually your doctor will choose a *broad spectrum antibiotic*, named for its capacity to kill many different kinds of bacteria. In a few days, when the lab can identify the exact organism, your antibiotic may be changed to one that is more specific for that organism.

Fine-Tuning the Antibiotic

To fight infections successfully you need the correct antibiotic at the correct dose for a long enough time to assure that the infection is gone. That is why your doctor and nurse will remind you to take all of the antibiotic prescribed, even though the signs and symptoms of infection seem to disappear after a day to two. Most antibiotic pills are prescribed for a week to ten days. More severe infections may require IV antibiotics for a few days, and then, depending on the organism and your response, you may be switched to pills, tablets, or capsules.

The dose of some antibiotics must be fine-tuned to be sure it is effective against the infection, but not harmful to your body. The doctor, therefore, needs to know the antibiotic's *peak* and *trough*. The peak is the greatest amount of medicine in your system (right after you receive it), and the trough is the least amount in your system (right before the next dose). To determine the peak and trough, your blood will be drawn twice, both before and after you get the medication. With this information, your doctor can adjust the dose to the right level for you.

Platelets

The cells in your blood that help to form a clot are called platelets. Platelets are produced in the bone marrow from a cell called a megakaryocyte.

Platelets help your body stop bleeding from knicks or cuts. They do that by collecting at the site of an injury and making the blood vessel constrict. Platelets then begin a series of chemical reactions that, along with other "clotting factors" in the liquid part of your blood, form a clot. After the vessel has healed and the clot has served its purpose, another series of chemical reactions cause the clot to dissolve so that the blood vessel is open again to carry blood.

Platelets are formed in large numbers, with up to 150,000 to 300,000 in each millimeter of blood. They live for about ten days in circulation. Chemotherapy slows down platelet production just as it slows down the production of all the other cells that are dividing frequently. The platelets in circulation are not affected because they aren't dividing, but formation of the megakaryocytes which will become new platelets may fall behind temporarily. The period of time when your platelet count is the lowest (the nadir) comes about ten to fourteen days after your chemotherapy. Then your platelet count rises during the next two weeks until it is back to normal.

What To Do When Your Platelet Count Is Low

Many people get through all their chemotherapy treatments without being in danger of serious bleeding because of lack of platelets. Mostly it is a matter of being more careful to avoid injury and paying more attention to any bruise or abrasion you get.

During the nadir, you may find that you bruise more easily or bleed slightly longer from a cut or after a blood test. Here are a few things to watch for:

- Check your skin all over for bruising or broken blood vessels. Check with your doctor if a bruise continues to increase in size or if you notice blood in your urine or bowel movements.

- Your mucous membranes are more likely to bleed as well. Even your normal toothbrushing and flossing may need to be altered during this time. Use a soft bristle brush and a more gentle technique.

Plasma

Electrolytes

Plasma is the fluid in which the red cells, white cells, and platelets circulate. It contains many substances that are essential for your body to function. Sodium, potassium, chloride, calcium, magnesium, and so on must be present in your body in specific amounts. That's because salts from these elements, when dissolved, can carry an electric charge that enables your heart, nerves, and muscles to work properly. These elements are called electrolytes.

Your kidneys help to regulate the balance of electrolytes by selectively eliminating or retaining these elements. For example, if you eat food that contains a high level of potassium, sodium, or calcium, your kidneys will keep what is needed and get rid of the excess. Chemotherapy treatments can temporarily affect your body's ability to keep a normal balance of electrolytes. Your doctor may therefore need to adjust the amount of electrolytes you get in your IV.

Proteins

There are also proteins in plasma. These are large molecules, such as albumen and globulin, whose presence controls the flow of fluid from the blood system to the cells. Low levels of albumen can occur with malnutrition. This may cause water and plasma to leak into the surrounding tissue, causing swelling (edema).

Enzymes

Your heart and liver contain unique enzymes. If these organs have been damaged (from a heart attack or from liver damage), then the enzyme specific to that organ can be detected at higher levels than normal in plasma. When the levels of these enzymes drop back to normal, it indicates that the organ is recovering.

Other Substances in Plasma

The levels of nitrogen, urea, and creatinine found in blood plasma indicate how well your kidneys are working. Since many chemotherapy drugs are excreted through your kidneys, your doctor will check the levels of these substances in your plasma before each treatment to determine the drugs and the doses that are safe and effective for you.

There are substances in plasma that are called *clotting factors*. They work with your platelets to form clots when needed and then work to dissolve the clots when they are no longer needed.

The amounts of glucose, protein, iron, and cholesterol in plasma can reflect your diet or digestion. An analysis of plasma can also provide early warning for diabetes, hormone imbalances, iron and vitamin deficiencies, or the risk of heart disease.

Testing plasma allows your doctor to check on how every organ is functioning. It is important to monitor not only how well the chemotherapy is working to kill cancer cells, but how the chemotherapy is affecting all the normal cells as well.

Tumor Markers

Research scientists are always looking for a simple blood test that will predict cancer at its earliest stage, as well as indicate how well the chemotherapy is working. This kind of test could also warn of recurrence long before there are any symptoms.

Although there is no current test that can accurately predict cancer's occurrence or cure, there are a number of substances in your blood whose presence at certain levels is associated with particular kinds of cancers. These substances are called *tumor markers*. Their levels tend to rise if the cancer is growing and drop when the cancer is destroyed.

An important drawback of tumor markers is that a rise in the tumor marker may not always be caused by cancer, but by another disease or condition. For instance, the level of the antigen alpha fetoprotein (AFP) is associated with liver cancer and ovarian cancer, but the level may also rise with hepatitis or pregnancy. A rise in the blood level of carcinoembryonic antigen (CEA) is associated with cancer of the colon, pancreas, breast, or intestines, but a rise in CEA may also occur with pancreatitis, inflammatory bowel disease, or emphysema. A rise in the enzyme prostatic acid phosphatase (PAP) is associated with cancer of the prostate, bone, or multiple myeloma. But a rise in PAP is also possible with osteoporosis.

In other words, tumor markers are not foolproof in being able to predict the presence or absence of cancer. But they are one of many tools your doctor has in following your progress.

Comparative X-rays, scans, and physical examinations, along with changes in your tumor markers, are all ways the doctor can tell how your treatment is progressing.

Interfacing with Other Health Care Professionals

Let your doctor know if you are planning any other medical treatments. Visits to the dentist, podiatrist, or chiropractor should be cleared by your oncologist first. During the period of time when you have fewer white cells or platelets than normal, you are more likely to bruise or bleed more easily and you are less resistant to infections. Your oncologist will advise you when other treatments are safe and the kind of precautions that other doctors need to take during this time. For the same reason, let other health professionals know that you are receiving chemotherapy so that they will consider this when planning and scheduling their treatments.

Coping

Blood tests are so common and useful in the diagnosis and treatment of diseases that medical people forget how stressful they may be for the patient. Here are some suggestions that may help you cope.

It helps if you can relax. If you are not in a panic, your veins are easier to find. Make sure that you are comfortable and your arm is well supported. When your arm stays still, the needle causes less pain.

If you can anticipate when the test will be done, you may want to ask for a warm blanket to wrap around your arms. The heat will make your veins swell and make it easier for the nurse or technician to take the blood sample.

When the test is over, apply pressure to the vein for at least five minutes. This is especially important if your platelet count is low and your body takes longer to form a clot. Applying pressure will minimize the amount of bruising and pain you have afterwards.

3

The IV Experience

Nobody likes needles. No one likes to extend his or her arm and await the tourniquet and the cold swab of alcohol. You pray that your veins will stand out and fear that the worried look of the technician indicates that you and your veins might be a problem. People who are receiving chemotherapy have to face that moment of truth many times during their treatment. Frequent blood tests are important to monitor your response to chemotherapy, the recovery of your immune system, the functioning of your kidneys, the presence of infection, and so on. Besides the blood tests, most chemotherapy drugs are given intravenously (in the vein, or IV for short). When medicine is sent into your vein, it is quickly distributed by the blood all through your body. Most chemotherapy drugs are not available in a form that you can swallow, because they may be damaging to the lining of your stomach or would be rendered less effective by the action of different gastrointestinal enzymes and secretions.

More About Veins

Veins and arteries are muscular tubes that respond by swelling or contracting in response to temperature, activity, or emotions. You can notice how prominent your veins get on a hot day or when you are playing baseball or kneading dough. You may have also noticed that your veins seem to disappear when you have been inactive, feel cold, or are anxious. Unfortunately, many people feel anxious when they are faced with needles while having an IV started or blood drawn. They find that their once prominent veins are nowhere to be seen. Closing down the blood circulation to arms and legs and shunting it to vital organs is a reflex that happens automatically when someone is afraid.

Fortunately, there are ways of getting veins to dilate and become more accessible. A tourniquet (the thick rubber band that gets wrapped around your upper arm) partially constricts the veins and traps some blood in the arms and hands, which makes your veins stand out. Warming your arms or flexing your muscles by clenching and unclenching your fist are other ways that your veins will fill with blood and stand out.

Good Veins and Bad Veins

The ease or the difficulty that a nurse may have in starting your IV depends on a number of factors. The condition of your blood vessels, both arteries and veins, reflects your general health and strength. Strong, young, muscular people tend to have strong, muscular blood vessels. Older people, as well as those who are ill or malnourished, have more fragile vessels. Frequent punctures and irritating medications such as antibiotics or chemotherapy can make veins temporarily less flexible and more tender and fragile. The skill and experience of the person approaching your veins is, of course, another factor. Starting an IV takes coordination, judgment, and skill. And the more experience that a person has, the fewer problems there will be with the procedure.

Which Vein?

Many different veins can be used to draw blood or start an IV if they are sufficiently large, close to the surface, and can be dilated by using a tourniquet. The tourniquet makes the veins easier to feel and see. After the blood sample has been collected or the IV started, the tourniquet is released and normal blood flow continues as before.

Blood samples are usually drawn from the large vein at the inside of your elbow. That vein, however, is rarely used in starting an IV because it would restrict the movement of your entire arm. In general, the veins in the back of your hand and the lower arm are best for IVs. They are visible and accessible, and the needle can be anchored (using tape) to prevent accidental removal without restricting your movement.

Needles

Short-Term IVs

The kind of needle used to start an IV depends on whether the IV will be used for a short time (just a few minutes) or over a longer period (several hours or days). Most chemotherapy given in the doctor's office flows into your blood in less than an hour. The kind of needle commonly used is a very thin metal needle, often called a "butterfly." It gets its name because the tabs on the side that the nurse holds onto during insertion look like the wings of a butterfly. Once the needle is in place, the wings are taped down to hold it still.

Right after insertion, you might see a little bit of blood flow back into the tubing attached to the needle. This indicates that the needle is inside the vein. Your nurse also verifies the correct placement of the IV by injecting a small amount of fluid into the needle. She can see that the fluid goes into the vein and not into the surrounding tissue. This shouldn't be painful, and once the needle is inserted and immobilized with tape there should be no further discomfort. Pain, burning, or swelling are all indications that the needle may not be in the vein or that the vein is leaking. You should tell your nurse immediately if you are having any of these symptoms.

Once the needle is secured and its position is verified, the medication will be given. It might be given through a syringe directly into the tubing of the butterfly needle. Or it may be diluted with a small amount of fluid from a bottle or plastic bag and dripped through tubing into your vein over a longer period of time. Once again, there should be no pain once the needle is secured.

Longer-Term IVs

If your treatment requires you to have an IV in your arm for a number of hours or longer, you need to be able to move around without dislodging the needle or damaging the vein. For longer term IVs, a thin, soft tube called an IV catheter is used. The catheter is about an inch long. At first, the catheter covers a thin steel needle. Once the catheter and needle are inserted into the vein, the steel needle is removed, leaving the soft, flexible catheter in place. The catheter is then secured by tape and a small dressing or bandaid is put over the place where the catheter enters your skin. This catheter may stay in place for up to three days.

As with the steel butterfly needle, the position in the vein is verified by the presence of blood in the tubing and by having a small amount of fluid rinsed through the catheter into the vein without causing pain or swelling of the surrounding tissue.

How Do You Cope?

Most nurses who work with chemotherapy have a lot of experience in starting IVs and are very skillful as well as relaxed and supportive. They know that most of their patients are anxious, especially when first getting chemotherapy. You are not the only one who feels this way.

People have different ways of coping with stressful situations. Some people cope by learning everything they can about a new experience. It helps them if they know what will happen, what it will look like, what it will feel like, and what will be expected of them. Others cope by withdrawing into themselves. They don't want a lot of detailed information, since it just makes them feel overwhelmed and more anxious. Distraction helps other people. They feel more relaxed if they can focus on something else—meditation, reading, watching TV, or talking.

Many people say it helps to have a close friend or relative with them for support. The support can be both physical (holding their hand, for instance) and emotional. Having someone to talk to you, distract you, read to you, or just sit quietly with you can make you feel safer and more comfortable in a stressful situation. If you do bring along a support person, be sure that the person knows what you want from him or her. Talk it over and be specific about what will help *you*. Do you want a quiet, calm presence, or would you rather have someone distract you with conversation and gossip?

Take some time to think about how you cope with stress— and then do all the things you can to support your coping style. Would it help you to be familiar with the environment? You can arrange to meet the nurses, to see the room, and even to see other patients who are receiving treatment. The nurses can tell you exactly what to expect and how long the process takes and give you answers to many questions.

While you are getting chemotherapy, your nurses can also be a source of support. Don't forget to communicate how they can help. Let them know what your needs are. You might say,

"It would help me to know exactly what I can expect. Please explain everything that is happening." Or you might say, "I brought a tape with me so I can just space out." Or, "I'd like my brother to stay with me."

Get comfortable. Because chemotherapy patients often have to sit still for an extended period of time, most clinics have comfortable recliner chairs for them. Loosen tight waistbands, ties, or collars. Bring a sweater or shawl or ask your nurse for a warm blanket if you get cold. Try to position the arm that has the IV comfortably. Since some chemotherapy medicines leave a metallic taste in your mouth (or your mouth may feel dry from the antinausea drugs or from anxiety), sucking on hard candy or chewing gum can be a help. The antinausea medications that you may get before your chemotherapy can also make you sleepy. If you feel that way, you may want to doze or listen to music on tape. Some clinics provide audio or video tapes or have a television that you can watch. Feel free to bring in your own tapes as well.

After your first treatment, your anxiety level should be much lower. The whole procedure, the environment, and the physical experience will be a little more familiar. You will also know more about what works and doesn't work to help you relax. Were you able to meditate, or was the room too distracting? Did your sister's endless chatter help pass the time, or was it annoying? Should you bring that murder mystery to read, or would you have preferred leafing through *People* magazine? You will also know the nurses better and feel more confident about their skill. And they will know you better and can begin to anticipate some of your individual physical and emotional needs.

Bags, Bottles, Tubing, and Pumps

IV fluids and medications flow through sterile tubing from a plastic bag or glass bottle. IVs flow by gravity, and the rate is adjusted with a roller clamp on the tube which controls the flow of fluid.

When the fluid or medicine needs to go at a very slow rate, it can be controlled with a special machine called an IV pump. An IV pump can be set at any rate. It also keeps track of how much fluid is left in the bag or bottle and can sense whether there is any resistance to the flow. Resistance indicates that the needle is dislodged or the tubing is kinked. The pump also keeps an electronic eye out for any air bubbles in the tubing, and it will make a loud beep to alert you and your nurse if there is a problem. The IV pump is attached to the pole holding the medicines and fluids. The pump plugs into an electrical outlet, but it has a built-in battery so that it can be unplugged for short periods of time and still continue to function.

Sometimes two different bags or bottles of fluid will be running simultaneously in an IV. For instance, you might have a *hydrating solution* which provides water and a small amount of salts and minerals. Another bag contains your chemotherapy, which is set to go in at a controlled rate over several hours or more. In addition, other bags might hold one or two IV medications to prevent nausea. These may be given both before your chemotherapy and at set intervals during your treatment. There may be times when your IV pole looks like a maze of bottles, tubes, and blinking lights, and you're not sure what is supposed to be dripping!

Your nurses will let you know what medicines you are getting, what they are for, and how they are likely to make you feel. For instance, some chemotherapy medicines are given with lots of hydrating fluids, and they will cause you to urinate frequently. Some antinausea medicines will make you feel sleepy or forgetful for a few hours. Knowing what to expect will make it all less frightening.

Staying Comfortable During Chemotherapy

During chemotherapy you should feel no pain or burning. Pain or burning from the IV indicates that the needle or catheter is not positioned properly in the vein and that it should be checked or changed. You should not feel nauseated, because you will probably be given medicines to prevent nausea. Most people get through their chemotherapy treatments without any discomfort, continuing to eat and drink normally. The next chapter on coping with nausea, will give you more information about the anti-nausea medicines and provide self-help tips to avoid this problem.

Staying comfortable in part depends on you. Only you can tell how you feel. You are the source of the essential information about what's happening inside your body. If you have nausea, stomach cramps, dizziness, or any other unusual symptom, let your nurses know so that they can contact your doctor and have the medicines changed. It might take some fine-tuning to get you the medications and doses that will keep you comfortable, but it can and should be done.

IV Problems

It is the moment that everyone fears. Your veins are small, fragile, or invisible. You endure several attempts at starting the IV, and both you and the nurse get more and more tense. What should you do?

Go for the pro. Successfully starting an IV depends a great deal on the skill and experience of the person doing it. And generally the most skillful people are the ones who do it frequently. In many hospitals there are special IV teams—nurses who are IV specialists. If you know that you are a "difficult start," you can ask for the IV specialist to see you, or you can ask for the most experienced nurse working on your floor or in the clinic. In time you will recognize some of the nurses and have more confidence in their ability. Just seeing a familiar face can help you relax, which helps your veins relax as well.

Stay calm. You have probably noticed that when you're anxious, your hands become cold and clammy. That's a normal reaction to fear. Unfortunately, anxiety works against you when you want the veins in your hands and arms to stand out. So anything you can do to lower your anxiety will probably help: deep breathing, having a supportive person with you, meditation, or even just a distraction. See Chapter 11 for more relaxation techniques.

Keep warm. Heat causes veins to dilate and fill with blood. That makes starting the IV easier. Your nurse may provide some form of heat for your arms, such as a warm blanket, heating pad, or a pan of warm water.

Keep drinking. Some people, afraid that they'll feel nauseated from their chemotherapy, don't eat or drink before their treatment. Since today's antinausea medications are so successful in preventing nausea, this really is not necessary. In fact, eating and drinking normally will keep your body fluids up and help make your IV easier to start. Your veins will be "fatter" with more blood if you don't let yourself become dehydrated.

What if Your IV Is Painful?

Sometimes, even if you've been careful not to disturb your IV, the catheter may become dislodged. Then the fluid or medicine, instead of flowing into your bloodstream, begins leaking into the tissue surrounding the vein. The affected area of your arm or hand might start to feel painful—tender, tight, or swollen. You may notice that your rings or watch feel tighter than usual. What should you do?

If you suspect that fluid is leaking out of the vein into the surrounding area, let your nurse know right away. It doesn't matter if it's day or night. The sooner the IV is removed and changed to another vein, the better. In the office or clinic, the nurse will be watching your vein and the flow of fluid carefully, especially if the chemotherapy medicine is being injected directly into the tubing connected to the needle. In the hospital, your nurse will check the flow of fluid as well as your arm and vein frequently. She or he will ask you if you have pain at the IV needle site. But don't wait to be asked. If you think there is a swelling or if you have any discomfort, then call right away.

Even if the catheter or needle is still in place and your vein is not leaking, your vein may feel irritated. Sometimes diluting the medicine with more fluid or slowing down the rate of the flow will help. Often, however, it is necessary for the nurse to change the IV to another vein (larger, if possible) so that the medicine can be swept along with a faster blood flow.

Monitoring the IV is clearly an important part of your treatment—and your nurse may not always be the first one to notice something. Even though she or he will often check your veins and the flow of medicine, it is always helpful for you to stay tuned in on your end.

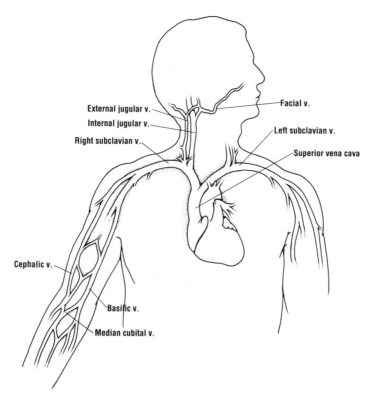

Figure 1. Veins of the arms and chest.

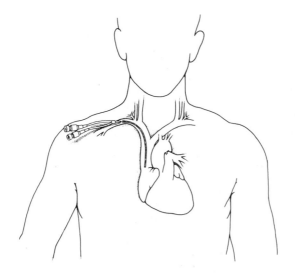

Figure 2. A central IV catheter.

Central Lines

Figure 1 shows the veins of the arms and upper chest. The arm veins are called peripheral veins, and the blood flow through them is relatively slow compared to the larger veins of the upper chest. All peripheral veins lead to larger and larger veins, which carry a faster blood flow on the way to the heart.

Central IV catheters are inserted into one of the large veins in the upper chest. They are called central IV lines because they go into the veins nearer the heart. They may be used for longer-term use when the veins in the hands and arms are fragile or difficult to find or if the kind of IV fluids needed would be damaging to the smaller peripheral veins.

This kind of catheter (shown in Figure 2) is inserted by a surgeon right in your hospital room using a local anesthetic. Usually the catheter emerges from the skin underneath the collar bone where it is sutured into place. Because the place where the catheter emerges from the skin is so close to where the catheter penetrates the central vein, there is added risk of infection entering the bloodstream. So the area where the catheter emerges must be kept sterile, and this requires special cleaning and dressings. Although this kind of IV is useful for patients while they are in the hospital, they are usually removed before anyone is discharged home.

Venous Access Devices

Most people receiving chemotherapy don't stay in the hospital for a long period of time—they may be in the hospital for a few days or receive their treatment in the office or clinic and not be hospitalized at all. Since central catheters are rarely used on an outpatient basis, chemotherapy treatments often involve multiple needle sticks for both blood tests and IVs. Never pleasant, this becomes especially problematic if your arm veins are fragile or small.

Fortunately, new products have been developed to overcome some of these IV problems. The new products are called *venous access devices* (VAD). They provide a way into the larger veins of the blood system, where the blood moves more quickly and the effects of medicines and fluid are not as irritating. Venous access devices eliminate the difficulty of trying to find veins and they make the process of starting IVs or taking a blood test quick and painless. They can also stay in place indefinitely, without interfering in your normal life at home.

Two kinds of devices are most frequently used at present. Both kinds use the large veins of the chest and are inserted by a surgeon during a minor outpatient surgical procedure that doesn't require an overnight hospital stay. Both kinds can be removed when chemotherapy treatment is over.

Tunneled Catheters

These IV lines enter a big vein in your upper body, usually near the collar bone. The catheter is advanced until the end of the catheter is situated near the heart, where the blood flow is fastest. The catheter can carry fluid, blood, and chemotherapy or other medicines, as well as provide blood for most blood tests. While similar to the central catheter described earlier, tunneled catheters don't emerge under your collar bone. Instead, they literally tunnel under the skin until they emerge from the front of your chest, about at the level of a second or third shirt button. Figure 3 shows approximately where the catheter comes out of your body. Its position makes it easier to care for the skin around the catheter. You can clean the area yourself, and the little dressing doesn't show with your clothes on. Because the place where the catheter enters the vein (up by your collar bone) is far away from where it emerges from your skin (midchest), there is less chance of the large vein getting infected.

When a tunneled catheter is inserted, the surgeon makes a small incision near your collar bone and threads the catheter

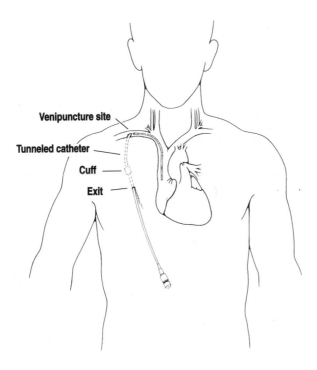

Venipuncture site

Tunneled catheter

Cuff

Exit

Figure 3. A tunneled catheter.

into a large central vein. Then he makes a tunnel under your skin from the vein towards the center of your chest. That is where the catheter emerges. Once the incision is healed and the minor swelling goes away, you should have no pain from the tunneled catheter.

Although there is only one tiny hole in your skin where the catheter emerges, the end of the catheter may split into two or more ends or *lumens*. The fluid going into one lumen does not mix with the fluid going into the other lumen. This arrangement enables someone to get more than one medication at a time when necessary.

A tunneled catheter means less needle sticks. The end of each lumen is capped off with a little rubber stopper. When the IV is started or a blood test is taken, the needle goes into the little rubber stopper, not into your skin!

The tunneled catheter requires daily cleaning at the place where the catheter comes out of your skin, and each lumen must be rinsed, according to the schedule your nurse gives you, with special fluid to prevent a blood clot from forming. People who have a tunneled catheter in place can shower normally after 72 hours. Then they clean the skin around the catheter by applying an antibiotic ointment and small dressing. If you have a tunneled catheter, your nurse will explain how to do the catheter care. She or he will give you time to practice rinsing the lumens, changing the caps, and keeping the skin around the catheter free from infection.

Implanted Vascular Access Devices

These catheters are also inserted into the large blood vessels of the upper chest. However, instead of emerging from the front of your chest, the catheter ends in a special device called a port that is implanted inside your skin (usually near your shoulder). Figure 4 shows an implanted port. The port is about the size of a half dollar, and the raised center area is about the size of a nickle. The center area consists of a thick, rubber-like plug that can be punctured with a special needle. Once the needle is secured and covered, it can be attached to a short length of IV tubing. Now the IV fluid, blood, or chemotherapy can flow into the port and through the catheter to the large veins.

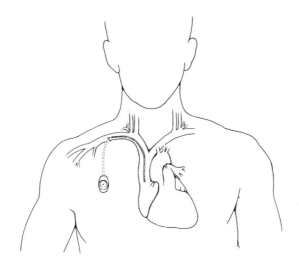

Figure 4. An implanted port.

When you first need to have an IV started or blood drawn, the nurse feels for the location of the raised center of the port, cleans the skin, and punctures through the skin straight into the center plug. Since the center is usually easy to feel, there should be no fishing around as there often is with regular IVs. Success is not dependent on your veins. The needle is held securely by the center plug and is much less likely to be dislodged. Once the needle is inserted and secured, the port can be used for all fluids, IV medications, or blood, and most blood tests can be drawn from the same port and the same needle without any other needle sticks. When your treatment is finished, the catheter is rinsed with a solution that will prevent a clot from forming, and the needle is removed. The rubber-like plug automatically seals itself so there is no bleeding from the port, as sometimes happens after a blood test from your vein.

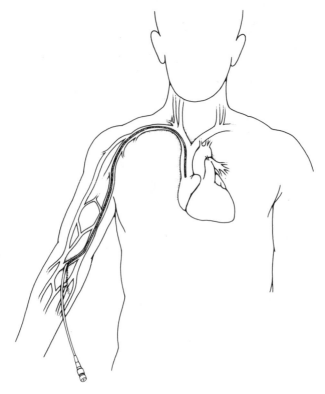

Figure 5. A peripheral inserted line (PIC).

The implanted port and catheter are put in by a surgeon during a minor surgical procedure. He makes a small incision, threads the catheter into the large vein, and then forms a little pocket for the port under the skin of your upper chest. Once the incision is healed and the tenderness and minor swelling go away, you should have no pain from the implanted port. Although you'll be able to feel the raised rubber center of the port, no part of the device is left outside of your skin. Once the incision is healed, you can bathe and even swim. No daily care is required, because your own skin protects the catheter from infection.

The implanted port and catheter can stay in place indefinitely. Usually the needle needs to be changed every seven days. Most people, even if their chemotherapy lasts for several days,

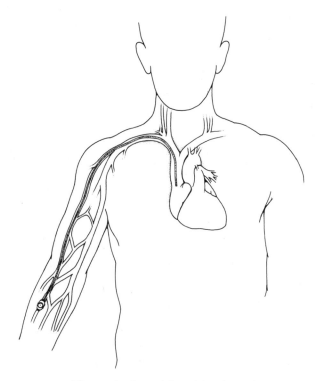

Figure 6. A peripheral implanted port.

are long gone from the hospital before the needle needs changing. The implanted port enables you to have most blood tests, IVs, and medications with only one needle stick a week.

Other IV Alternatives

New devices and techniques are always being developed to make the IV experience less traumatic, less painful, and more dependable. An alternative method for getting to the big veins uses a very long catheter which is inserted in an arm vein and then threaded up until it gets to the larger vein in the upper chest. This device (shown in Figure 5) is called a peripheral inserted central line (PIC) because the catheter is inserted peripherally (into your arm), but travels to a large central vein (in your chest). The end of the catheter emerges from your arm and requires special cleaning and dressings to prevent infection.

There is also a small port (shown in Figure 6) that can be implanted in your arm. As with the PIC, a long catheter then travels from your arm into a large vein of your upper chest. The advantage of this device over the PIC is that the catheter never emerges from your skin. It ends at the implanted port and remains sterile. It requires no special cleaning or dressing and, like the implanted chest port, only a single needle stick to gain access to the blood system.

Which One Is Right for Me?

Not everyone will need a tunneled catheter or an implanted port. There are many, many people who complete their chemotherapy treatment and blood tests without needing any kind of device. Their veins can tolerate the kind of medications and fluid they need. Although it's never pleasant to have IVs started or blood drawn, they get through it without major problems.

If you do need a venous access device, you and your doctor will discuss the risks and benefits of each one. Your doctor will consider the kind of chemotherapy you need, your anatomy, and your preference. You will be able to see what each device looks like and perhaps talk to someone who has one.

Although it's not easy to face the minor surgery that's needed to have a VAD put in your body, once it is in place many people experience it as a great relief. Their IVs are easily started, blood tests are easily obtained, and their arms and hands are freer while they are getting treatment.

Getting Through It

Nobody likes needles! For many people, a good deal of dread and fear about getting chemotherapy is associated with the frequent blood tests and IVs. They may feel out of control when their veins won't cooperate and IV starts become difficult.

In time you'll find your own unique ways of relaxing and coping during this stressful period. Hopefully, you'll come to trust the skill and support of the people who are caring for you. Just knowing what to expect, what is happening, and what it will feel like can make it all less overwhelming.

4

Coping with Nausea

Of the possible side effects of chemotherapy, people often say they dread feeling nauseated and vomiting the most. They may have known someone who received chemotherapy treatments and who suffered severe nausea without effective medication. Or they may recall a time during their own life when they were nauseated and remember how debilitating it was.

It is a misconception that people who receive chemotherapy suffer continuous and unrelieved nausea and vomiting. First, not all chemotherapy drugs cause severe nausea. Some drugs given in low doses may cause mild nausea or no nausea at all. Second, this problem, even for the most nauseating drugs, usually lasts for a limited amount of time (from two to eight hours for most drugs). Third, there has been an enormous amount of research toward developing effective treatments to prevent or aggressively relieve the nausea associated with chemotherapy.

Preventing this side effect is very important. If you are able to stay well nourished, feel good, and maintain your activities, you will be more able and willing to complete your treatment. This is possible only if side effects like nausea and vomiting can be controlled.

Not All Chemotherapy Causes Nausea

Every chemotherapy drug has been rated as to its "emetic potential"— the chances that it will cause you to feel nauseated or to vomit. Some rarely cause nausea (meaning that less than 30 percent of people taking the drug feel that symptom). Some are considered only moderately nauseating. And then there are drugs that are very likely to make you feel nauseated (meaning that 90 percent of the people report the symptom). So right from the beginning, your doctor can tell you if nausea is likely to be a problem.

Another factor that may determine how nauseated you may feel is the dose. A chemotherapy drug may not cause nausea at a low dose, but it may cause the problem at higher doses or when given in combination with other more nauseating drugs.

Finally, there are always individual differences in how people react to any medication. Some people are just more likely to feel nauseated, just as there are some people who are more likely to suffer morning sickness, motion sickness, or sea sickness. Your doctor may try to predict how much of a problem nausea will be, but you may be less or more nauseated than expected. The key is to work with your doctor and nurse to determine the type and the amount of antinausea medication you need to prevent or minimize this problem.

Bear in mind that whether or not you become nauseated from any chemotherapy drug does *not* indicate if the chemotherapy is working. And when you get medications to prevent or relieve nausea, it does not make the chemotherapy less effective.

What Causes Nausea?

The feeling of nausea and the act of vomiting are not really caused by your stomach. There is actually an area in your brain that, when stimulated, causes these feelings. It is called the *chemoreceptor trigger zone* (CTZ), and it lies in the center of your brain. This area may be stimulated by a number of different events. The CTZ may be stimulated by a feeling of fullness in your stomach (from too much pizza and beer), or it may be stimulated by dizziness (sea sickness or motion sickness). Certain sights, smells, or thoughts may cause nausea as well. Some people may feel nauseated and even vomit from anxiety, fear, stage fright, the sight of blood, unpleasant smells, or the thought of getting an injection. The CTZ center is also sensitive to chemicals in your body. Some chemotherapy drugs make your body release other chemicals, such as dopamine or serotonin, which stimulate the CTZ.

The stimulus that triggers nausea can come from different places in your body—from the stomach, the inner ear, sensations, and thought—as well as from chemicals. To prevent or relieve nausea, different drugs work in different ways. Some drugs prevent nausea by blocking the body's release of histamine, dopamine, or serotonin, so that the CTZ will not be stimulated. Some drugs speed up the action of the stomach and intestines to make the stomach empty quickly so that there is less fullness to stimulate the CTZ. Other medications help you relax and even sleep through the period of time when you are most likely to feel nauseated.

The goals of taking antinausea medication are to prevent nausea, improve your ability to eat and drink after chemotherapy, and allow you to continue your normal activities as soon as possible.

Types of Antinausea Medicines and How They Work

The following group of drugs is commonly used to prevent nausea during chemotherapy. The generic name is given first, followed by the brand names that may be more familiar to you. Next comes a general discussion of how the drug works and some side effects to watch out for.

Prochlorperazine (Compazine). This drug has been the mainstay of antinausea treatment for over twenty years. It acts in the chemoreceptor trigger zone by blocking dopamine receptors. Dopamine is released by the body in response to some chemotherapy drugs and causes nausea. Compazine can be used alone for preventing nausea when getting mildly nauseating chemotherapy drugs. It is available in many forms, including a pill, a long-acting capsule, a rectal suppository, or an injection in the muscle or vein.

Side effects to watch for are drowsiness (don't drive) and low blood pressure (usually only a problem if given by vein). Prochlorperazine may also cause an uncomfortable jitteriness or restlessness. This reaction is called *akathisia* and goes away if you take a mild tranquilizer such as diazepam or lorazepam (Valium or Ativan). You may also experience a tightness in the muscles of your jaw or face. This is called *dystonia* and is easily reversed by taking a mild antihistamine, such as diphenhydramine (Benadryl). If you are having these side effects, be sure to call your doctor to see if he or she wants you to change to a different medication or to take additional medications to counteract these symptoms.

Metoclopramide (Reglan). Reglan works in three ways to prevent nausea. It helps the stomach empty quickly and it also blocks dopamine in the CTZ. In high doses, it blocks serotonin. It is taken in smaller doses by pill and in larger doses by vein. It is very helpful in preventing nausea with even the most nauseating chemotherapy medicines.

Side effects to watch for at higher doses are drowsiness (don't drive) and diarrhea or abdominal cramping (it speeds up the intestinal tract). It may cause restlessness and anxiety, as well as tight facial muscles, similar to prochlorperazine (Compazine). If you are having these side effects, you should check with your doctor to see if you need an antidiarrhea medication or other medications to reverse the side effects as described in the section on prochlorperazine. When high doses of Reglan are used in the hospital, the medications to reverse Reglan's side effects are often given simultaneously to prevent these symptoms from occurring at all. Other dopamine-blocking drugs work in similar ways. Each will have some variation in its antinausea effects as well as its side effects. If one drug is not effective to prevent nausea or causes side effects that are a problem, another drug may be substituted.

Ondansetron (Zofran). This is a relatively new antinausea drug used since 1991. It works by preventing serotonin (a chemical released by your body in response to chemotherapy) from getting through to the CTZ and causing nausea. Ondansetron is very effective in preventing nausea from even the most nauseating chemotherapy drugs. It is usually given in the vein before chemotherapy and is repeated in 4 and 8 hours. It is also effective at a higher dose given just once prior to chemotherapy. If the chemotherapy drug causes nausea that lasts more than 24 hours, ondansetron can be given the next few days as well, although it seems to work better during the early phase of nausea.

Another advantage of ondansetron is that is does not have the side effects of some of the other antinausea medicines. It will not make you sleepy and does not cause the restlessness or muscle stiffness that prochlorperazine (Compazine) or metoclopramide (Reglan) have been known to cause. The most common side effect associated with ondansetron is a mild headache or constipation.

Lorazepam (Ativan). This drug is a tranquilizer in the same family as Valium. It doesn't block dopamine at the CTZ or speed up the digestive tract. It works in the brain by making you relaxed, forgetful, and sleepy. It is sometimes used alone, but often in combination with other antinausea drugs when people are getting moderately to highly nauseating chemotherapy medicines. You can take this drug by mouth or by injection in the muscle or vein. It is also easily absorbed through the mucous membranes and so it can be dissolved under the tongue. This is particularly convenient if you are vomiting and have difficulty keeping pills down.

The side effects to watch for are sedation and forgetfulness. Do not drive when taking this drug. You may find that you do not remember events or conversations you have had while taking Ativan. It may also cause a mild lowering of blood pressure, weakness, or unsteadiness. Call your doctor if these side effects are a problem. You may need to use a smaller dose, take it less often, or change to a different medication.

Steroids (Dexamethazone—Decadron, Hexadrol). It is not known exactly how steroids work to prevent nausea. It's possible that they block the chemicals released by the body (in response to chemotherapy) from getting through to the CTZ and therefore make it less likely that you will feel nauseated. They are usually given in combination with other antinausea medicines. Since you take them only for a few doses, you don't have to worry about the side effects of long term use of steroids. These drugs are usually given by vein.

The side effects to watch for are water retention, restlessness, confusion, and euphoria (feeling high). Also, if given too rapidly in the vein, steroids may cause a temporary feeling of itchiness or burning in the vaginal or rectal area that lasts only a few minutes and goes away on its own. People who have diabetes need to be aware that steroids can cause a temporary elevation in blood sugar.

Combination of drugs. As you can tell from the preceding list of medications, different antinausea drugs work in different ways. One drug prevents the chemotherapy from affecting the CTZ. Another speeds up the digestive system. Another helps to lower anxiety, making you relaxed and sleepy. Your doctor may recommend a combination of antinausea medicines to most effectively prevent nausea.

Start by taking the medication in the dose and frequency recommended. For instance, your doctor might recommend taking Compazine every four to six hours. Be alert to any side effects that may occur, and notify your doctor or nurse as soon as possible if you are having any problems. Remember, everyone has his or her own unique responses to chemotherapy and to the antinausea medicines. Your doctor needs your feedback to make adjustments in the plan so that it works for you. You may need to change to a different medication. You may need to change the schedule of the dose or frequency of the medication, or you may need to add another medication to counteract a bothersome side effect.

Nausea from Anticipation

Another kind of nausea is not caused by the chemotherapy drug, but by anticipation. People who suffer *unrelieved* nausea after several chemotherapy treatments begin automatically to associate chemotherapy with feeling nauseated. This is a *conditioned response* to a strongly unpleasant experience. As a result, anything associated with chemotherapy may trigger this reaction— the ride to the office or hospital, the sight of the nurse or the IV tubing, the smell of the alcohol, and so on. This phenomenon of feeling nauseated without a physiological reason is called *anticipatory nausea and vomiting* (ANV). The best treatment for ANV is prevention. If you don't suffer significant nausea after your chemotherapy, then you are not likely to anticipate feeling nauseated with the next treatment.

Anxiety also contributes to anticipatory nausea. Some people avoid pretreatment jitters and nausea by taking an antinausea medication even before they leave the house (or, if they have to drive themselves, they may take the pill immediately after arriving for their appointment). The medication that seems to work best for ANV is Ativan, but anything that allows you to relax will help prevent nausea. The following are a few suggestions.

Progressive muscle relaxation (PMR) is a way of counteracting anxiety. You can learn to relax all the muscles of your body, visualize pleasant scenes or sounds, and psychologically remove yourself from a stressful environment. See Chapter 11 on relaxation and stress reduction for more information on PMR.

Systematic desensitization has been used successfully for this problem. This technique is a kind of counter-conditioning used in treatment of anxiety and phobia. After you learn to relax your body, various anxiety-provoking scenes associated with chemotherapy are visualized starting from the least anxiety provoking to the scariest. For instance, you might start by visualizing driving to the clinic or doctor's office for your chemotherapy. You learn to relax while visualizing this scene. Then you slowly work up to the scarier scenes (such as having the IV started and the medication going in). When you learn to relax your body while visualizing the whole procedure from beginning to end, you may find that you are less anxious and less nauseated. Complete instructions for systematic desensitization are given in Chapter 11.

In addition to PMR and systematic desensitization, other relaxation techniques may prove useful to relieve anticipatory nausea. Deep breathing, relaxation imagery, autogenics, and self-hypnosis are excellent relaxers and are fully explained in Chapter 11.

Sometimes just bringing a book or a magazine to glance through may distract you. Some people find that bringing a friend to sit and chat or read to them during the treatment is very helpful to lower their anxiety and lessen their chances of anticipatory nausea.

The Importance of Fluid

Everything that you take by mouth (food, fluids, medication, and so on) eventually enters your bloodstream, where it circulates through your entire body. It is finally removed from the blood by the liver or kidneys and is usually eliminated in the urine. Some chemotherapy drugs can cause direct damage to the bladder or kidneys if they are not eliminated fast enough. That is why it is so important to drink enough fluid after you've had chemotherapy. The more fluid you take in, the easier it is for your body to break down the chemical by-products of the chemotherapy and eliminate them.

One of the dangers of continuous nausea and vomiting is that it makes it difficult to take fluids by mouth. If you are in the hospital for your chemotherapy treatment, you will receive fluid directly in your vein so that it is not so important for you to drink a lot. But when you are at home after your treatment or after a stay in the hospital, it is especially important to control nausea so that you can drink. If you are too nauseated to drink, you may become dry or dehydrated. When you are dry, the nausea may get worse. The result is a vicious cycle: unrelieved nausea causes dehydration, which intensifies the nausea. Preventing that cycle is essential.

What Is Dehydration?

If you have not been able to drink because of nausea or if you've been vomiting a great deal, you will feel dry. Your mouth and lips will be dry and may be flaky or cracked. Your blood pressure may be lower than usual, and so you may feel dizzy when first standing up. (Note that since dry mouth and slight dizziness may also be side effects of some antinausea medicines, those symptoms may not necessarily mean that you are dehydrated.) Your body will try to hold onto all the fluid it can, so you will notice that you are urinating less frequently and that the volume of urine is less than usual. Your urine may also appear darker because it is more concentrated. You may notice that your weight is down several pounds from before you had your chemotherapy. These are all signs of dehydration.

What To Do If You Are Becoming Dehydrated

Be sure that you are taking the antinausea medication prescribed. If you are vomiting and cannot keep pills down, call your doctor for advice. You may need to take a rectal suppository or some other form of medication that you can tolerate.

After taking the medications, wait about half an hour and then try taking sips of fluid. Any kind of fluid is fine—water, tea, popsicles, or broth. Drink a small amount frequently (try half a cup every half hour).

Keep track of how much fluid you are taking and how often you are vomiting, as well as how often you are urinating. If you are still nauseated, call your doctor and tell him or her:

1. How much fluid you drank in the last 24 hours.

2. How often and approximately how much you have vomited in the last 24 hours.

3. What antinausea medicines have been prescribed, whether or not you have taken them, and what problems, if any, they have caused.

4. How often and approximately how much you have urinated and if your urine appears dark. (Some chemotherapy medicines will discolor your urine for a few hours, so that it may be difficult to tell if your urine appears darker than normal due to dehydration.)

5. If you have lost weight since getting your chemotherapy.

6. If your mouth, lips, and skin feel dry.

7. If and when you feel dizzy (all the time or just when first rising from a sitting or lying down position).

8. Be sure to tell the doctor if you have any other relevant problems. For instance:

   • If you have a fever (take your temperature before calling).

   • If you have pain—where, how long it lasts, what makes it better, what makes it worse.

   • If you are a diabetic, check your blood sugar before calling.

   • If you have missed taking other medications because of the nausea or vomiting (heart or blood pressure medications, anticonvulsants, pain medication, hormones, and so on).

Your doctor may want you to come into the office or clinic to check your blood pressure and for blood tests to see how dehydrated you have become. It may be necessary to give you extra fluid by vein as well as make changes in the antinausea medicines you take at home. Dehydration is a temporary condition that is usually corrected quickly with replaced fluid and medicines.

Here are some suggestions for the hours after you receive chemotherapy to prevent dehydration.

1. When you first get home, take the antinausea medication at the dose and times recommended *before* you experience nausea. That way you can continue to take fluids, wash the chemotherapy by-products out of your body, and feel better sooner.

2. Follow the set schedule of medications as recommended by your doctor or nurse. That will keep you covered

during the hours when you're most likely to have problems.

3. If your nausea is not relieved by the medication or you're having problems with side effects, contact your doctor or nurse for advice. They may advise you to change medication, change its dose or frequency, add another medication that will relieve your symptoms or counteract side effects, or change the form of the medication—you might need medication by rectal suppository until you're able to keep fluid down.

Step-by-Step Hints

Before Chemotherapy

It is not necessary to have an empty stomach before getting chemotherapy. Staying well nourished and well hydrated (drinking lots of fluids) will help you feel stronger and help your body eliminate the chemotherapy by-products more quickly. Eat and drink regularly until about two hours before your treatment. Eat foods that are easily digested (high carbohydrate, low fat). Stay away from spicy food or food that will give you a lingering aftertaste that may make you feel nauseated later (onions, garlic, and so on). Your doctor may want you to take antinausea medicine before coming to the hospital.

During Chemotherapy

Do whatever you can to lower your anxiety. Bring a book, a music tape, or a friend. Some antinausea medicine might make you feel sleepy, so sleeping through your treatment might be possible. Wear comfortable clothes, loosen you belt or tie, and bring a sweater or ask for a blanket if you feel cold. Sometimes chemotherapy drugs leave a metallic or unpleasant taste in your mouth. Sucking on hard candy or chewing gum might help.

After Chemotherapy

Medications. Take the antinausea medications as prescribed. Do *not* wait to feel nauseated to take the medications. Your aim is to get through the high-risk hours and not feel nauseated at all.

Food and fluids. Eat small amounts, more frequently. Avoid feeling overfull. Eat bland foods (mashed potatoes, cottage cheese, toast, sherbet, crackers).

You may be very sensitive to the smells of food. Foods that are served cold or at room temperature have less aroma. Stay out of the kitchen as much as possible. Prepare foods for yourself or the family that are quick and easy with minimal sights or smells that may be upsetting to you.

If you are diabetic, you have to be careful that your insulin dose is appropriate for how much you are eating. You might need to check your blood sugar several times that day to make sure it is not getting too low or too high. Your doctor may want to adjust your insulin doses until you're able to eat normally.

Sometimes sweet juices are hard to tolerate after chemotherapy. If that's true for you, try lemonade, broth, club soda, or ice water. Try mixing a little juice with mineral water. You might need to try several different kinds of tastes before you discover what works best.

It is most important to take fluids. Don't worry if at first you don't feel like eating solid foods. Try popsicles, tea, juices, soup, ice. Drink fluids before and after eating solid food. Drinking *with* your meal may make you feel overfull and bloated. Drink *small* amounts of fluids *frequently* to avoid feeling too full.

Rinse your mouth or brush your teeth after eating to avoid lingering tastes that may be nauseating.

Activities. Fresh air and mild physical activity help prevent nausea. Take a walk or sit on the porch or by an open window. Distractions may help. Go to the movies, read a book, talk to a friend, listen to music, play cards, and so on.

Sleep. Some antinausea medications may make you sleepy. Let yourself sleep through the high-risk hours. If you are supposed to take some medication on a set schedule around the clock, you may want to set the alarm clock so that you can wake up, take the medication, and then go back to sleep. If you are not taking medication in the middle of the night, take it when you first wake up, before you get out of bed and start moving around.

Relaxation. If you are feeling anxious, relaxing may be easier said than done. There are a number of audio and video tapes that you may find useful in getting you through relaxation exercises. They can help you clear your mind and relax every muscle in your body. You may find that the tension you are holding in your face and jaw or in your shoulders or abdominal muscles is adding to your anxiety or feelings of queasiness. Some tapes provide peaceful and relaxing images and music. After you practice with these tapes for a period of time, you may be able to relax yourself very quickly with or without the tape any time you feel tense or anxious. You can also make your own tape with the relaxation script provided in Chapter 12 of this book.

Self-talk. The things you say to yourself can help you cope or cause you more stress. Many of these thoughts are unconscious and so automatic that you may not even be aware of them. Pay attention and try to tune into what you may be saying to yourself that is increasing your stress and worries about nausea (or any other scary symptom). It may help to write these scary thoughts down. This makes them more conscious and more manageable. It also allows you to argue against them and replace these anxiety-provoking thoughts with thoughts that are supportive, accurate, and focused on coping.

Your anxiety-producing thoughts may sound like this:

- I can't stand it—this is too much.

- I feel so helpless, there is nothing I can do.

- The antinausea medicine isn't working—nothing will help.

- I'll never feel any better.

You can replace these with supportive thoughts that help you cope:

- I can get through this—this discomfort will only last a few hours.

- If this medicine isn't working to relieve my nausea, there are other medicines that I can try.

- The chemotherapy is effective, no matter how nauseated I feel.

- I'm learning how my body reacts to chemotherapy and to the antinausea medicines.

- I am in charge—I can take the medicine that I need to feel better.

- It's okay to sleep and let the hours pass.

- The kids (or husband or job) are taken care of for now. Right now I can pay attention to me and take care of myself.

- I know how to relax, distract myself, and feel better.

- I know that _____ is here for me if I need him or her.

Write down your own coping thoughts. When you find your anxiety rising, tune into what you are silently saying to yourself and talk back, using the coping statements that help you feel better.

Thought-stopping techniques can literally block negative thoughts before they make you anxious. Thought stopping is explained in detail in chapter 11.

Nausea and vomiting can be very debilitating, both physically and psychologically. Fortunately, there are strong and effective medications and relaxation techniques that really work. Lots of people get through their chemotherapy treatment with minimal nausea or no nausea at all. That is the goal—to get through this time and remain comfortable, well nourished, and able to do the normal activities of your life as soon as possible. Preventing or relieving the side effects of chemotherapy, especially nausea, is a very important part of your treatment.

5

Coping with Other Digestion Problems

When people think about chemotherapy and its side effects, nausea and vomiting are the symptoms that most frequently come to mind. But other parts of the digestive system can be affected by chemotherapy as well. Unlike nausea, which is associated with the period of time immediately following treatment, other digestive side effects are not apparent until a week or two later. Here's why.

Chemotherapy affects cells that are frequently dividing, and these include the cells lining your entire digestive system. Normally cells that are old or dying are shed and replaced by new cells. But if there is a delay in the replacement of old cells because of the effects of chemotherapy, then you can develop digestive problems such as sore mouth and throat and diarrhea.

This chapter will discuss these and other side effects that cause temporary changes in the digestive system, why they occur, and what you can do to feel better.

Parts of the Digestive System

In order to visualize the way food travels through your body, you might think of a large tube. This tube starts at your mouth and ends at your rectum. The mouth is the place where the digestion of food and fluids starts. When you chew, the food is mixed with saliva which begins to break down the food into substances the body can use.

When you swallow, the food and fluids travel down a long straight section of the tube called the esophagus which connects to your stomach. Once in the stomach, food is further broken down by the mechanical action of muscles churning and the chemical action of the acidic digestive enzymes found there.

The partially digested food moves from your stomach into the small intestines, which are approximately 21 feet long. Because they are so long and the space in your abdomen is fairly compact, the intestines wind back and forth in your abdominal cavity like a ribbon. It is in the small intestines that most of the nutrients are absorbed into your bloodstream.

What remains of food after digestion are waste products. These move into the large intestines (also known as the colon). The colon is about five feet in length and ends with your rectum. As the waste products move through the large intestines, fluid is absorbed. By the time the waste products have traveled through the entire colon and are ready to be eliminated from your body, the stool is no longer liquid, but a formed solid.

Mouth and Throat Problems

During the months while you are receiving chemotherapy, there may be times when your mouth and throat become sore. The soreness may start with a feeling of hypersensitivity to sour or spicy tastes and some redness or swelling of your gums, cheeks, palate, or throat. There may be open areas similar to cold sores on the sides. Brushing your teeth, rinsing with a mouthwash, eating, or even swallowing may be very painful.

Your doctor or nurse may call this condition *mucositis* or *stomatitis*. Mucositis means an inflammation of the mucous membranes of your gastrointestinal system, while stomatitis is an inflammation of the mucous linings of your mouth. Both terms describe the problem that may occur when the surface layer of cells lining your mouth and throat are not replaced as quickly as usual because of the chemotherapy. If you have inflammation or sores in your esophagus, it's called *esophagitis*.

Some chemotherapy agents such as 5-Fluorouracil (5-FU) are more likely than others to cause this problem. As with any side effect caused by chemotherapy drugs, the chance of developing the problem and the severity of the problem if it does occur are related not only to the type of medication, but also to the dose and your general health and age.

Not everyone who receives chemotherapy will develop mucositis, but it is good to be able to recognize the problem early and know what to do. While this condition is painful and uncomfortable, it will improve fairly quickly as the cells recuperate. However, during the time you are experiencing mucositis, there are a number of things that you can try to feel better, promote healing, and prevent infection.

Self-Help Suggestions for Mouth and Throat Sores

Keeping your mouth clean and comfortable. First, the cleaner your mouth is, the better it will feel. Brushing your teeth or dentures and rinsing your mouth within thirty minutes after meals is very important. If your doctor or nurse says that your platelet count is low, you will be more susceptible to bleeding and bruising. In this case, you should use a soft toothbrush to avoid traumatizing the tissues of your mouth. If you wet your toothbrush in hot water it will soften the bristles even more. An alternative to a soft toothbrush is a sponge-tipped swab. You can wet the swab and use it to gently clean your mouth as well as to stimulate your mucous membranes. One word of caution regarding the sponge-tipped swab—it is not as effective as a toothbrush in removing debris or plaque from your teeth. When your platelet count returns to a level high enough to prevent bleeding, go back to using your toothbrush. If your platelet count is low, do not use floss or a strong stream of water from a water-jet, as these could also cause bleeding.

Try to keep your lips moist by using a lip gel or even a light layer of Vaseline. Most lip gels or balms have an oil base which will protect your lips for several hours. Soon you will notice that the dry skin is noticeably softer and that the cracks are beginning to heal as well.

Mouth rinses. In addition to using a tartar control toothpaste, rinse and gargle with a diluted solution of baking soda. Use one teaspoon of baking soda mixed into a glass of water. The baking soda solution cleans, promotes healing, and lowers the acidity in your mouth. This helps if you have vomited and some of the acid in your stomach has come up into your mouth. Rinsing with baking soda solution will help to neutralize the effects of acidic debris on your tender oral tissues.

If you have sore mouth, avoid using commercial mouthwashes or products which contain alcohol or glycerine. Both will dry your mouth tissues even more and make the soreness worse.

Eating hints. When your mouth or throat are sore, avoid foods which are hot or spicy. Foods which contain chili powder or pepper (like some Mexican or Thai dishes) may cause more pain. Avoid drinks that are hot or make your mouth sting. Citrus juice (such as orange or grapefruit juice) may be a problem because it is acidic. Cool bland fluids (apple juice, herbal teas) will be more soothing to your mouth and throat.

Yeast Infections

Whenever the normal balance of organisms that naturally live in and on your body changes, you are more likely to develop a yeast infection. Many women know that when they are taking antibiotics they are more likely to develop vaginal yeast infections. The normal balance of organisms that live in your mouth can also be changed because of chemotherapy or a change in your nutrition.

If you notice that there are white patches on the insides of your cheeks or along the gum line, you may have a yeast infection in your mouth (also known as *thrush*). Call your doctor or nurse so that he or she can prescribe an antifungal medication (such as Nystatin or Mycostatin) to eliminate the problem.

If the medication comes as a lozenge, let it melt slowly in your mouth so that it can cover all your mouth surfaces as well as your throat. If you have difficulty with the lozenges because your mouth is very dry or sore, then tell the doctor so that he or she can order the medication in a liquid form. You can take about a teaspoon of the liquid and swish it around in your mouth so that it covers all of the surfaces of your cheeks and gums. Then let it roll back into your throat and gargle with it so that it can also coat your throat. You can then either swallow it or spit it out. Since your esophagus may also be sore or infected, swallowing the antifungal solution will allow it to coat this area as well.

Another way to take the antifungal solution is to measure out your doses into ice cube trays and freeze them. Then, when it's time to take your next dose of Nystatin, you can pop a "Nystatin-sicle" in your mouth. As it melts, it can provide soothing coolness and comfort to your tissues.

Mouth Pain

Most people are able to cope with the short period of time that their mouths and throats are sore without too much difficulty. But sometimes mouth pain is so severe that it interferes with your ability to eat or drink. When you have severe pain in other parts of your body, you would naturally try to protect that part by resting it until it was no longer hurting. When your mouth is sore, that remedy is not possible, since you must continue to take fluids and nourishment orally. If your mouth pain becomes severe, notify your physician as soon as possible. You may need to rinse your mouth with a special medication that will numb the tissues and relieve the pain before you can eat or clean your mouth. But be aware that if you use medicine that numbs your throat, you should wait at least thirty minutes before eating or drinking, because the medicine can suppress your natural gag reflex. If the gag reflex is not working, food or liquid can more easily be swallowed the "wrong way" and be inhaled into your lungs.

If your mouth pain is so severe that you cannot eat or drink enough fluids to prevent dehydration, you may need to have IV fluids and pain medication for a few days until you are feeling better.

Taste Changes

After chemotherapy, some foods which previously tasted good to you may now have a different, even unpleasant flavor. For example, red meat may taste bitter, or sweet foods may taste more or less sweet then you are used to. The reason for this is that your taste buds may be temporarily altered by chemotherapy. So even foods that you crave may taste different in an unpleasant way.

Taste changes are usually not permanent. Even after the high doses of chemotherapy given for bone marrow transplantation, people say that their sense of taste eventually returns to normal. But give it time; it may take several months. In the meantime, here are some ways you can deal with the problem.

Cleaning your mouth by brushing and rinsing with the baking soda solution before meals can help. When your mouth is clean and moist, flavors of foods may be more distinct. If your mouth feels like it is filled with cotton, the taste of food will not be as pleasant.

Experiment with eating foods with various kinds of flavors to see which ones taste good to you and which ones to avoid. Try eating foods with different textures to make eating more enjoyable when your sense of taste is altered. Chapter 6 has many suggestions about how to deal with taste changes. You can also ask your doctor to recommend a nutritionist to help you find foods that are more appealing so you can stay well nourished even while you are experiencing this problem.

Food Aversions

During chemotherapy you can get very turned off to some foods. If you eat and immediately feel nauseated, the food you have just eaten becomes mentally associated with the feeling of being sick. You may then feel nauseated or vomit when you try to eat that same food again. Therefore, when you are feeling nauseated, do not eat all of your favorite foods in an attempt to increase your appetite. If you do this, you may find yourself without any favorite foods left.

Anorexia

Anorexia is a term which describes not feeling like eating or not being hungry. After your chemotherapy treatments, the food you eat may take a long time to move through the digestive tract. If the food is "sitting" in your stomach, you will have a feeling of fullness and eating may become difficult. With or without the feeling of fullness, your appetite may wane. A large plate of food (even something you might like) can make you feel overwhelmed or discouraged.

One way of managing anorexia is to try to eat smaller meals more frequently. Instead of three large meals, some people eat five to six meals, spaced throughout the day.

Preparing a meal can also contribute to anorexia. If you are having problems with nausea or fatigue, just the thought of making a meal may be enough to keep you from trying to eat. Freezing single-size portions of foods you like may help. On days when you do not feel up to cooking, you can heat up a frozen meal with minimal effort. Try stimulating your appetite with foods prepared and served attractively. If you can tolerate more flavorful foods, try eating foods which are spicy, sweet, or sour so that they are more interesting.

If anorexia is affecting you to the point that you are losing weight, your doctor may prescribe medications that can stimulate your appetite. If the problem is compounded by problems of nausea or slow movement of food through your digestive tract, other medications may be helpful as well. A dietician or nutritionist may offer other suggestions so that you can maintain good nutrition until your appetite returns to normal. Chapter 6 has many suggestions about how to spark your appetite.

Intestinal Problems

Diarrhea

When you have diarrhea, food moves through your large intestines so quickly that the water is not able to be absorbed normally. Therefore, your bowel movements are more liquid and more frequent. This problem can be very distressing and disruptive to your normal routine and can cause severe fluid loss and imbalances in the salts and minerals your body needs. There are a number of different reasons that people getting chemotherapy can develop diarrhea.

Effects of chemotherapy. Chemotherapy damages the cells in the intestinal tract that are dividing frequently. When that happens, the body responds by trying to remove the damaged tissue as quickly as possible. The rhythmic movement of your intestines (peristalsis) speeds up, and anything in the intestines moves out rapidly in the form of liquid stools. Diarrhea caused by the effects of chemotherapy will improve when the intestinal lining heals.

Effects of medications. Diarrhea may also be caused by medications given to prevent nausea. Metoclopramide (Reglan) increases the movement of food and fluid through the digestive tract. This relieves the feeling of food sitting in the pit of your stomach. One problem with this increased movement is that it sometimes becomes diarrhea.

Effects of infection. Diarrhea can also be caused by infection. Chemotherapy suppresses your immune system, and so you have fewer white cells to fight infection. As a result, bacteria that wouldn't bother you when your immune system is functioning normally may be able to attack when your defenses are temporarily weakened by the chemotherapy.

What To Do When You Have Diarrhea

If you are having frequent loose stools, let your doctor or nurse know right away. Keep track of the frequency and approximate amount of your stools. You may be asked to collect a small amount of stool for the lab so that it can be tested for infection. If the cause of diarrhea is not infectious, your doctor may prescribe an antidiarrhea medicine to slow down your bowels. If an antinausea medicine is causing the problem, your doctor may recommend that you decrease the dose or frequency, or you may be switched to another antinausea medicine.

When you have diarrhea, you may lose so much fluid that you can become dehydrated. Along with the fluid, you lose important minerals (especially potassium). If severe diarrhea goes untreated, you may experience other signs of dehydration such as feeling dizzy or weak. Your kidneys will make less urine in an attempt to hold onto fluid and, as a result, may have difficulty removing waste products.

For all of these reasons, it is important to maintain your fluid intake and replace lost minerals. Try slowly sipping small amounts of fluids such as fruit juices and nectars, soups or Gatorade (a drink specially formulated to replace lost electrolytes in your body). Since drinking very cold fluids can irritate your intestines and cause more discomfort, try drinking moderately cool or lukewarm fluids. If you feel like drinking sodas such as ginger ale, it's best to let the "fizz" out first so that you won't feel bloated. (The carbonation in the soda can also irritate your throat as it goes down.) If you are at home, weigh yourself and keep a record of the amounts and types of fluids you are drinking so that your doctor will have information to help determine if you are becoming dehydrated.

Antidiarrhea Medications

Diarrhea can be your body's way of getting rid of the organism causing the infection or toxic products produced by the organism. Just as it is important to remove a splinter from your finger so that it can heal, moving the infected stool out quickly is the best way of promoting healing of the intestines. Stopping or slowing down the diarrhea allows the infection to stay longer and causes more damage. If the stool sample shows that you have an infection, you will first be given antibiotics to cure the infection, before you are given any medication to slow down the diarrhea.

If you do not have an infection, you can use antidiarrhea medicines. Lomotil or Immodium will slow down the rhythmic movement of your intestine and allow liquid to be absorbed from the stool, producing firmer bowel movements.

Constipation

Constipation means a decrease in the usual frequency of bowel movements. When you are constipated, the stool stays in your intestines longer, and so it may become very dry and hard. There are a number of reasons you could become constipated during this time. Some are directly related to the chemotherapy, some are not.

Anything that slows the movement of your intestines will cause constipation, and some chemotherapy drugs such as Vincristine can cause your intestines to slow down. You can also become constipated if you are taking pain medicines frequently, because they too will slow the digestive tract. If you are less active than usual, the normal rhythm of your intestines is slowed. If you are not eating or drinking as much as you usually do because of nausea, fatigue, or a poor appetite, that can make you dehydrated and cause constipation as well.

What To Do To Prevent Constipation

Fluids. Just increasing the amount of fluids you drink will help your bowel movements become softer. Warm, noncaffeinated liquids such as herbal teas, fruit juices, or prune juice are helpful to keep your intestines moving and prevent constipation.

Food. High-fiber foods such as raw vegetables and beans will increase the bulk in your stools and stimulate the intestines to move. But if you increase the fiber in your diet, be sure to increase the fluid you drink. Since the job of the intestines is to absorb fluid as well as nutrients, if you increase the bulk without increasing the fluid you will become more constipated than before. See Chapter 6 for more information about food choices for a high-fiber diet.

Activity. There are a number of reasons why you may be less active while on chemotherapy. Your usual routines might be changed drastically because of the necessity of keeping appointments at the clinic or hospital or at the lab for diagnostic tests. Besides, you may just feel a lot more fatigued than usual during this time. Pain medications or antinausea medication may also make you sleepy and less active. Or you may not have energy because you are not eating or sleeping as well. But even if you are not up to your usual exercise program, some activity may help relieve constipation. Even walking each day in the fresh air will make a difference.

Laxatives, stool softeners, and enemas. Although many medications are available to treat constipation, check with your doctor before taking any to make sure that you are using the right one for you.

Stool softeners work by combining or mixing with the stool to make it more oily or more liquid. Colace, Ducosate Sodium, or DSS are examples of stool softeners. Oil-based suppositories such as Glycerine work in much the same way.

Laxatives stimulate the intestines to move the stool along at a faster rate and thus prevent the stool from getting too hard or dry. Drugs such as castor oil, Cascara, or Dulcolax increase the movement in the intestines by irritation. The intestines move faster in an attempt to remove the irritating substance out of the body sooner.

Metamucil or Citrucel contain indigestible products such as bran or methyl cellulose, which increase the volume of the stool in your intestines. When your stool has more bulk, the feeling of fullness in your rectum stimulates the urge to have a bowel movement. Fruits or vegetables work the same way because the indigestible portions of those foods contribute to the bulk of your stool.

Milk of Magnesia or magnesium citrate contain nonabsorbable salts which help retain fluid in your stool. With the increase in fluid, the stool is bulkier and thus stimulates the urge to have a bowel movement.

Enemas work to stimulate your intestines by irritating them or by increasing the volume of substances in them.

Be sure to check with your doctor before using any medication rectally. During the times when your white count or platelet count are low, you could risk infection or trauma by using an enema or suppository. Prolonged use of laxatives or enemas may also inhibit your body's natural ability to have a "normal" bowel movement.

Coping

You can see that there are many side effects other than nausea which can affect the digestive system during chemotherapy. What is important to remember is that all of these side effects can be managed. Your doctor has many tools at his or her disposal, and there is much that you can do to increase your own comfort as well.

6

Maintaining Good Nutrition

by Barbara Yost, R.D.

Eating a balanced diet is an important part of good health. During chemotherapy, eating well is especially important. A balanced diet provides the proteins, fats, carbohydrates, vitamins, and minerals to give you energy, repair normal tissue, and fight infection. Eating well supports your body and helps normal cells recover quickly.

But food provides more than just the fuel for your daily activities. Eating special foods can also be a way you nurture yourself. And sharing meals is a way of socializing with others. People eat out in restaurants to celebrate or relax. Preparing food for others is one way that people show their love and concern.

When your ability to eat normally is changed, even temporarily, it can affect more than your nutrition. It can affect your sense of self and your ability to enjoy the pleasurable sensations and activities that occur around the experience of eating.

How Does Chemotherapy Affect the Digestive System?

From your mouth to your large intestine, your digestive system is lined with rapidly dividing cells that are vulnerable to the effects of chemotherapy. Chemotherapy can cause a change in appetite, alter your sense of taste, and cause nausea, diarrhea, or constipation. These side effects can make it hard to eat a balanced diet.

The side effects of chemotherapy and their severity depend on the particular medicines and dosages taken and individual sensitivities. You may also be taking other medications that can cause digestive problems. For instance, pain medicines can cause constipation, and some antinausea medicines can cause diarrhea.

Certain side effects are more likely at certain times. Nausea or fatigue may be problems for the first day or so after your treatment. Diarrhea may be a problem a week or so later. The explanations for these differences are covered in Chapters 4 and 5.

Because your symptoms may change, your eating strategies may need to change as well. After several cycles of chemotherapy, you will have a much better idea of the difficulty (if any) you may have maintaining a healthy diet. This chapter will give you some idea of the problems that may arise and some suggestions to help you overcome them.

Cancer, Chemotherapy, and Weight Loss

Cancer is often associated with a profound loss of weight. As cancer cells are rapidly growing and dividing, they use the vitamins, minerals, proteins, and calories that the rest of your body needs. They sometimes also release chemicals that speed up the body's use of these nutrients or suppress your appetite. Cancer cells can also interfere with your ability to chew, swallow, or digest your food normally. And your appetite can be poor due to taste changes, fatigue, or the stress of being ill.

Staying well nourished and maintaining your weight while you are receiving chemotherapy is particularly important to your recovery. Your doctor and nurse will weigh you at each visit and monitor your weight carefully as an indication of your ability to tolerate the chemotherapy. Think of food as part of your healing—one feature of your recovery over which you have some control.

Your goal is to eat the amount and balance of nutrients required to support your exceptional needs over the course of your treatment. Start by following your personal food preferences, tastes, and routines. You know your likes and dislikes best and have a good idea of food you can and cannot tolerate. The more you "normalize" your eating and your activities around food, the better you'll feel and the more successful you'll be in meeting your goal.

Anticancer Diets

The challenge while getting chemotherapy is to eat enough calories to maintain your weight and provide energy to fight infection and recover from the effects of your treatments. You've probably read about diets that protect you from cancer: high fiber, increased vitamins A, C, and E, more broccoli and sweet potatoes, less total fat. But when you are dealing with the problems of nausea, poor appetite, or feeling full quickly, some of the features of an anticancer diet are inappropriate. For example, foods higher in fat provide more calories for less volume than low-fat foods, or, when you are having diarrhea, you won't want to be eating broccoli.

Aim to keep a five to ten pound weight range around your usual weight. If you don't have a scale, buy or borrow one to keep track of how well you are maintaining your weight within that range.

During the months of your chemotherapy treatment, your weight will fluctuate. There will be days when you won't have much of an appetite and will want to eat light. On other days, you'll eat normally. The few pounds that you lose at one point can be made up when you are feeling better. Follow the suggestions at the end of this chapter to boost the number of calories in your diet during the catch-up phase.

Stimulate Your Appetite

Even though your appetite may be poor, there are things that you can do to stimulate your desire for food.

Go to a market or delicatessen and search out foods that appeal to you. Look through cookbooks and magazines for ideas for tasty foods.

Eating out can stimulate your appetite. In a restaurant you have the opportunity to choose from an enticing variety of foods, and you don't have to do the shopping, preparation, or cleanup.

Vary the surroundings where you eat. Eat on the front porch or in the garden. Use a cloth napkin or table cloth for another change. Make mealtime a treat to all your senses. Listen to relaxing music, dim the lights, brighten the table with flowers. Remind yourself to stay calm and unhurried.

Give thought to how the foods look on the plate. A variety of colors, textures, aromas, and shapes makes a meal interesting. Add a garnish. Set a colorful place.

Eating with other people and sharing conversation can also be stimulating. Induce a good friend to come once a week with a prepared meal for the two of you to share. Read or watch TV or an old movie while you eat.

Light exercise can also increase your appetite. Walking in the fresh air before a meal may help you feel hungry and more energetic. If you can't get out of the house, light housekeeping or craft work can be stimulating to your appetite.

If you feel full too quickly, try eating frequent small meals. Become a grazer—eat a bite or two every few minutes. Keep snacks handy, in different rooms of your house. You will eat more if food is readily available. Eat whenever you are hungry, at meal times and between meals too.

You may find food more attractive if you serve yourself small portions. A huge pile of food on a plate or a giant glass of beverage can be a turn-off if you are not feeling particularly hungry.

Small Amount—Big Calories

When you can't eat as much as you usually do, increase the calories in the food that you do eat. Calories are a measure of the energy a food provides. Normally you need about 12 to 14 calories per pound to maintain your weight. Healing from surgery or recovering from the effects of chemotherapy takes extra energy, so you need even more calories.

One apple has about 80 calories; one slice of apple pie has about 400. If your appetite is poor and the pie appeals to you, eat the pie and get five times as many calories. Instead of drinking a plain glass of milk, make a milk shake with added ice cream. If a liquid diet is all you can tolerate, make the liquids high in calories. Use a blender to make sherbet shakes. Add an egg. Make your cereal or cocoa with milk or half-and-half instead of water. Add cream to your soups. Spread mayonnaise, peanut butter, or cream cheese on bread. Smother vegetables with cheese or cream sauces. Drink eggnog with your meals.

The chart at the end of this chapter contains sample menus that are high in calories and protein and nutritious as well.

Weight Gain

Some people gain weight during the months of chemotherapy. An increase can be caused by a number of things, but unusual weight gain should always be evaluated by your doctor.

Eating to control nausea. Some people experience mild nausea for a few days after chemotherapy. Avoiding an empty stomach sometimes helps overcome this discomfort. Women who are having morning sickness in early pregnancy also find this method of controlling nausea effective. If you are snacking continuously between meals, cut down on the amount of food you eat at regular meal times to keep your weight in the normal range. Also check with your doctor about alternative antinausea medications which may be more effective in controlling your nausea when you are having this problem.

Steroids. Steroids (prednisone, dexamethasone, etc.) are sometimes part of your chemotherapy treatment. A side effect of taking large doses of steroids over an extended period is that they change your metabolism—the rate at which you use calories. Some people may even develop a form of diabetes during the time they are taking high-dose steroids, so that they are required to eat a calorie-controlled diet or take insulin during this time. Steroids can also stimulate your appetite as well as cause you to retain fluids. This too can cause weight gain.

Retaining fluids. Another reason for your weight gain is that your body may be collecting fluid in an abnormal way. Cancer can cause fluid to accumulate in your lungs or abdomen. Pressure on a large blood vessel can cause swelling in your legs. If your weight is going up without any apparent reason, check with your doctor. Let him or her know how much weight you have gained since your last appointment. Also mention if your ankles are swollen, if you are feeling short of breath, or if your abdomen seems larger (or your waist band seems tighter) than usual.

Large volumes of fluid by IV over several days may cause a temporary weight gain. Your kidneys will usually filter out the excess fluid, but sometimes it takes a while to catch up. Your doctor may prescribe a diuretic to help your body eliminate the excess.

Changes in Taste

Tasting food is essential to our enjoyment of eating. Even as children, we have our favorite foods and flavors. When things taste different, it can be very disorienting. People on chemotherapy sometimes experience a temporary change in their sense of taste caused by medicines entering the saliva and altering the taste of food. Temporary changes in the mucous membranes of your mouth may have the same effect.

People report that sweets taste more or less sweet during chemotherapy. Red meat such as beef or lamb may taste bitter, and foods that are usually bitter may taste more so. A common complaint is that foods taste salty or metallic or that the flavors of food are reduced.

Here are some suggestions that you can use to cope. If foods taste dull, try cooking the food in ways that heighten the flavor. Cook with wine or use salad dressings or strong seasonings. Smooth, bland foods may taste chalky or like paste. Garlic, onions, lemon, mint, and oregano are a few of the strong flavors that will help give food more taste and make it more appealing.

When your sense of taste is altered, use other senses to enhance meals. Keep appealing dishes covered until served, allowing the burst of aroma to tantalize you when the food is uncovered. Serve foods with distinctive textures. Crisp, smooth, crunchy, and chewy foods will stimulate your mouth. Eating some foods cold or frozen may increase their appeal.

Temporarily eliminate offending foods from your diet. If you have lost your desire to eat meat, substitute other high-protein foods such as eggs, cheese, milk, dried beans, or nuts. Replace salty foods with the salt-free variety. If something tastes too sweet, find a less sweet substitute. Return foods to your diet when they no longer taste "funny."

Bitterness is sometimes helped by eliminating metal pots or pans when cooking. Most food can be cooked in ovenproof glass or in plastic in the microwave. Marinate red meat in soy sauce, fruit juice, or wine before cooking to reduce bitterness. Chicken, turkey, and ham may still appeal to you when red meats do not.

If food tastes metallic, try sucking on lemon drops or a tart fruit candy before meals. Rinsing your mouth may also help decrease a metallic taste.

Any liquid nutritional supplements that you use to boost calories may taste better cold or over ice. You can get rid of any "vitamin" smell by drinking from a covered cup through a straw.

Be creative. Discover the flavors that you enjoy or that "come through" by experimentation. Find the foods that appeal to you and prepare them in ways that spark your appetite.

Nausea

Chemotherapy and nausea are so often associated that many people fear that nausea is an inevitable side effect of their treatment. This is not true. The chance of developing nausea depends on the specific drug you take, its dose, and your particular reaction to it.

Prevention of nausea for those who are likely to develop the problem is essential. A number of the drugs that are prescribed for this purpose are often given even before the chemotherapy is given. Most people, including those getting large doses of the most nausea-inducing drugs, are usually comfortable and able to eat normally, even on the day of their treatment.

In the hospital, nurses will give you nausea-preventing drugs (called antiemetics) at intervals so you don't experience the problem. The success of this approach can make it easy to forget that your comfort is dependent on taking the antiemetic. Some people feel so well in the hospital that they wait until they feel nauseated before taking these drugs at home. The trick is to avoid the problem so you don't run the risk of getting dehydrated, developing food aversions, or "anticipatory" nausea. Read Chapter 4 for descriptions of the drugs available to prevent nausea, an explanation of how they work, and suggestions for how to eat before and after your chemotherapy treatments.

Sometimes the feeling of nausea is mild, and people find that eating frequently settles the stomach. Morning nausea can be avoided by keeping crackers and juice by the bed so you can eat before getting up.

If you don't feel like eating solid food, it is especially important to drink fluids so you don't become dehydrated. Drink small amounts of cool, clear beverages frequently (every 15 to 30 minutes) if possible.

When you know that putting anything in your stomach will make you vomit, wait. Don't try to eat or drink until the vomiting is under control. Vomiting will further deplete you of fluids and electrolytes. You may first have to take an antiemetic medicine by rectal suppository. If you continue to vomit and cannot keep anything down, call your doctor. You may need to take fluids and antiemetics by IV to prevent dehydration.

Once vomiting is under control, try small amounts of water (one sip every ten minutes, advancing to one to two tablespoons every twenty to thirty minutes). If you keep this down for an hour, increase clear liquids slowly and gradually work up to a small, bland meal (like chicken and rice soup and crackers). If you can tolerate this meal, advance towards a normal diet. When you are hungry and think that you can hold food down, choose bland, low-fat foods that are easily digested. Sometimes eating foods cold will prevent their odors from stimulating nausea.

Rest after eating and focus on deep, natural breathing. Here are some foods that are easily tolerated when you are feeling nauseated.

- Apple or grape juice
- Fruit nectars (peach, apricot, guava)
- Bottled fruit-and-water blends
- Cold melon
- Fruit smoothies

- Sherbet
- Popsicles
- Jello
- Apple sauce
- Oatmeal or Cream of Wheat
- Canned fruits
- Angel food cake

Dry Mouth

Chemotherapy's effect on the mucous membranes in your mouth can cause a temporary decrease in the amount of saliva you produce. Additional drugs such as antiemetics or pain medicines can also dry your mouth. Your mouth may feel so dry that it is hard to eat. A dry mouth can cause foods to taste strange and make chewing and swallowing uncomfortable.

Dry foods like bread or meat can make the problem worse. When you are not producing enough saliva to mix with your food and allow it to be swallowed easily, add gravy or sauces. Dip cookies in tea to make them moist. Cook vegetables until soft or even puree them.

If your mouth is dry, drink lots of fluids, both with and between meals. Keep a cup of juice, tea, or broth close by and sip often, swishing the liquid around before swallowing to moisten all surfaces of your mouth.

If your mouth is not sore, try tart or sweet beverages or foods (like lemonade) to stimulate your mouth's production of saliva. Chewing gum or sucking on hard candy or popsicles also stimulates saliva.

If your lips are also dry, use lip salves to keep them moistened. Saliva also helps clean your teeth. Avoid dental problems by brushing your teeth and rinsing your mouth often, especially after eating.

Thick, sticky saliva may be a problem too. It can build up, especially during the night, and add to the problem of early morning nausea. Rinsing your mouth with warm water before eating will thin your saliva. Drinking hot beverages, such as tea with lemon, or sucking on hard candy will stimulate saliva and loosen thick mucus.

Try these foods when your mouth is dry or if you have thick, sticky saliva.

- Thin, hot cereal
- Warm lemonade
- Melon
- Diluted fruit juice
- Popsicles or fruit ices
- Thin, broth-based soups (chicken and rice, beef noodle)
- Cooked fish or chicken in broth
- Blended vegetables or fruit diluted to a thin consistency

Sore Mouth and Throat

Your mouth and throat may feel sore and sensitive for a period of time during your chemotherapy treatments. Chapter 5 discusses this problem and what to do to prevent and treat the soreness and infections if they occur.

When your mouth is sore, chewing and swallowing can be painful. Some foods are especially irritating and should be avoided. Other foods are soothing. Try these suggestions if your mouth is sore.

Eat cool, smooth foods to reduce discomfort. Stay away from spicy, hot, or salty foods or acid foods like citrus fruits and juices.

Avoid rough, coarse, or dry foods like raw vegetables, granola, or hard toast. Let hot foods cool down before eating or drinking them.

Puree food in a blender or food processor. Baby food is also bland, smooth, and easy to tolerate.

Use a straw to drink liquids, to deliver fluid to the back of your throat and avoid sore areas.

Nutritional supplements are a good source of high-calorie, high-protein, nonacid liquid. You can buy products like Ensure Plus or Sustacal in a drug store or mix your own by adding milk to Instant Breakfast. Look for brands that have more than 300 calories per cup of prepared liquid. A chart at the end of this chapter compares some popular nutritional supplements.

Here are some other cool, soft, nonacid, nonspicy foods that you can try.

- Milk shakes, nectars, grape juice, popsicles, jello
- Canned or soft fruits (bananas, applesauce, melon)
- Cottage cheese, mashed potatoes, macaroni and cheese
- Scrambled eggs, cooked cereal
- Pureed vegetables and meats (like baby food)
- Custard, pudding, milk toast, ice cream

Diarrhea

Diarrhea causes the food and liquids you have eaten to pass through your bowel so quickly that water cannot be absorbed from your digestive system normally. When this happens, you lose more than just water, you lose salts and minerals essential to the functioning of other body systems. Too much fluid loss may result in severe dehydration and weakness.

Diarrhea can be caused by a number of conditions including infection, food sensitivities, and antibiotics or other medications. Medications that prevent nausea sometimes work by speeding up the movement of food through the digestive system, which can also cause diarrhea.

The cells in your intestinal tract are vulnerable to chemotherapy medications. A week or so after your treatment you may develop diarrhea, because these frequently dividing cells are not being replaced at the usual rate. You are also more likely to develop intestinal infections at this time.

Unrelieved diarrhea can be a serious problem. Call your doctor if it continues. She or he may want to test a sample of your diarrhea for infection or prescribe a medication to slow down your intestines. If you have become dehydrated, you may need to replace fluid and salts through IV fluids.

Sometimes your doctor will want you to rest your bowel by eating only clear liquids for a day or two. Make up for the loss of calories when you are eating normally again to stay within your target weight range.

When you are having diarrhea, you want to eat low-fiber, nonirritating foods. Here are some suggestions.

During this time avoid caffeine (coffee, strong tea, chocolate), as it may aggravate the diarrhea. Also avoid greasy, fatty, or fried foods, raw fruits and vegetables, strong spices, carbonated beverages, and milk products.

Try the BRAT diet: Bananas, Rice, Applesauce, and weak herbal Tea, all of which are easily digested and unlikely to stimulate more diarrhea. The foods suggested for soothing a sore mouth (with the exception of milk products) are also good choices when you have diarrhea.

Eat small, frequent meals and drink plenty of liquids at room temperature between meals to make up for lost fluids. You need lots of extra sodium and potassium to replace what you are losing to diarrhea. Canned soups are high in sodium and easily digested. Bananas, apricot nectar, or mashed potatoes will supply potassium. Mix mashed potatoes with chicken broth to make a creamy, milk-free soup that provides fluid, sodium, and potassium. Also try these foods:

- Yogurt
- Smooth peanut butter
- White bread
- Noodles

- Tender meats
- Fish

Constipation

Constipation occurs when your intestines slow down and you have fewer bowel movements. Since the food lingers longer than usual in your bowel, more water than usual is absorbed, and your stool becomes hard and dry. People who are constipated feel uncomfortably full, which can reduce their appetite. Pain medications often cause constipation, and lack of activity makes it worse. See Chapter 5 for more information about this problem.

The key is to prevent constipation. Your doctor may prescribe a stool softener, which holds water in the digestive system. Other medications stimulate the bowel, so that food will pass more quickly through it.

If you're constipated, drink plenty of liquids between meals, get daily exercise if possible, and eat a high-fiber diet. Also try these foods to prevent constipation:

- Whole grain—whole wheat, bran flakes, wheat bran
- Raw fruits and vegetables
- Dried fruits, prunes, prune juice

Fatigue

You may find that there are periods of time, especially the first few days after your chemotherapy treatments, when you feel extremely fatigued. If you are the cook in your family, you will have to plan ahead so that you can get the rest as well as the nutrition you need when you are feeling tired. Here are some ways you can simplify things around mealtime.

Prepare meals in advance and freeze meal-size portions that can be easily thawed and warmed up in the microwave or oven. Casseroles are especially good, because they combine protein and carbohydrates in one dish. Store-bought frozen entrees, pizza, or take-out food can also be an easy dinner for your family when you are too tired to cook.

Ask a friend or family member to cook a dinner for you and your family when you are feeling tired. Help them by preparing a list of foods and spices that you would enjoy or would prefer to avoid.

Keep foods on hand that need very little preparation. Yogurt, canned fruit, canned soups, crackers, custard, eggs, and cheese are easy to prepare and are still nutritious. Keep snack food nearby (on the TV or on your nightstand) so that you can reach for it easily without having to get up.

Minimize cleanup whenever possible. Use paper plates and cups more frequently and use cooking containers that can go from the freezer to the oven to the table so that there is less to wash. Ask others to help. Even young children can clear the table or stack the dishes in the sink.

Chapter 9 has more information and suggestions about how to cope with the problems of fatigue.

Other Resources

Here are several additional sources of information to help you plan, shop, and cook food during this time when your dietary needs and problems are changing.

S. Aker and P. Lenssen. *A Guide to Good Nutrition During and After Chemotherapy.* 3rd Edition, 1988. This describes ways to eat while you are experiencing different side effects of chemotherapy. Write to Clinical Nutrition Program, Division of Clinical Research, Fred Hutchinson Cancer Research Center, 1124 Columbia Street, Seattle, WA 98104.

Eating Hints: Recipes and Hints for Better Nutrition During Cancer Treatment. U.S. Department of Health and Human Services, National Cancer Institute, 1992. Free. Call 1-800-422-6237.

Eating Smart. American Cancer Society, 1987. This covers dietary recommendations that minimize cancer risk for the general population, and is useful after chemotherapy. Free. Call 1-800-227-2345.

M. Mora and E. Potts. *CHOICES: Realistic Alternatives in Cancer Treatment.* Avon Books, 1987. A self-help cancer information book covering all kinds of cancer and cancer treatments.

Nutrition, An Ally In Cancer Therapy. Ross Laboratories. 1989. This tells you different ways to use nutritional supplements. Write to Ross Laboratories, Columbus, Ohio 43216.

About the Author

Barbara J. Yost is a Registered Dietition and Certified Nutrition Support Dietician. She graduated in Dietetics from the University of California, Berkeley, and completed a Masters Degree at Tuft's University. Barbara has a wide range of experience in the nutrition field, having taught nurses and worked in an outpatient clinic with all ages. Currently, she works at Alta Bates Medical Center in Berkeley, California with cancer patients and patients in Intensive Care.

Sample Menus

Regular, Healthy Menu	Bland, Soft Menu (For sore mouth, delicate digestion)	High-Calorie, High-Protein Menu (For weight gain)	Light Diet Menu Therapy (Use for chemotherapy or nausea days)
Breakfast Bran flakes Non-fat milk Cantaloupe Whole wheat toast* Butter, Jam*	**Breakfast** Cream of Wheat Poached egg Instant breakfast Apricot nectar	**Breakfast** Eggs, sausage Pancakes Syrup, Butter Orange juice Instant breakfast	**Breakfast** Herbal tea Cold melon Cream of Wheat Sugar
Lunch Black bean soup Turkey sandwich on whole wheat bread Raw carrots and cherry tomatoes Buttermilk	**Lunch** Cream of potato soup Cottage cheese and canned fruit Milk shake	**Lunch** Cheeseburger French fries Milk shake Apple pie	**Lunch** Cottage cheese and fresh fruit Herbal tea Sugar Crackers Popsicle
Dinner Spaghetti with meat sauce Tossed salad with broccoli, Oil and vinegar*, Garlic bread, Sherbet	**Dinner** Macaroni and cheese Cooked carrots Tapioca pudding Apple juice	**Dinner** Fried chicken Coleslaw Potato salad Biscuit and butter Apricot nectar	**Dinner** Apple juice Chicken and rice soup Jello
Snack Ideas Fresh fruit Dried fruit Raw vegetables Yogurt Bread Fruit juice	**Snack Ideas** Nectar Pudding Pound cake Bananas Mild cheese Canned fruit Ice cream	**Snack Ideas** Ice cream, Cake, Cookies Milk, Fresh fruit salad with sour cream and brown sugar Candy Nutritional supplements	**Snack Ideas** Nonacid juices Nectars Soups Frozen yogurt
*Omit these items if small or female	*You may need to divide food into 6 or more small meals to be comfortable*	*Don't fill up on fruits and vegetables*	*Make up for any weight lost as soon as you feel better.*

*Omit meat if vegetarian; use soy milk or supplements if lactose intolerant

Liquid Nutritional Supplements Comparison Table

Sample Items	Approximate		Added Vitamins and Minerals	Lactose?
	Calories/cup	Protein/cup		
Whole milk	160	8 grams	A, D	Yes
"Double" strength milk	250	16 grams	A, D	Yes
Instant Breakfast type powders	280	15 grams	Yes	Yes
Ensure, Isocal, Resource, Attain, Replete	250	9 grams	Yes	No
Ensure Plus, Resource Plus, Nutren 1.5, Sustacal HC	350	13 grams	Yes	No
McDonald's milkshake	350	9 grams	No	Yes
Haagen Daz, Ben and Jerry's ice creams	500	4 grams	No	Yes

Major Nutrients, Their Sources, and Functions

Nutrient and Safe/Recommended Intake	Important Sources	Functions in the Human Body
PROTEIN 1/2 gram/pound	Meat, fish, poultry, eggs, dairy, nuts, legumes, seeds	Build and repair body tissues; make enzymes and antibodies
FAT less than 30% of calories	Butter, cream, oil, bacon, margarine, nuts, mayonnaise	Concentrated calories for energy; supplies essential fatty acids, carries soluble vitamins A, D, E, K
VITAMIN A RDA: 5000 IU	Liver, egg yolk, milk. Beta carotene: apricots, cantalope, mangos, dark green and deep yellow vegetables	Promotes smooth skin, healthy mucous membranes; essential for growth; protects against night blindness; antioxidant
VITAMIN D RDA: 400 IU	Vitamin D fortified milk, brewer's yeast, fish liver oil, synthesized by action of sunlight on skin	Absorbs dietary calcium and phosphorus; for strong bones and teeth
VITAMIN E RDA: 18 IU	Wheat germ oil, vegetable oil, leafy green vegetables, whole grain cereals, liver	Helps prevent destruction of vitamin A and C; helps prevent some infantile anemias; antioxidant
THIAMINE (B1) RDA: 1.5 MG	Brewer's yeast, wheat germ, pork, beef, liver, whole grain products, legumes, enriched flour	To use carbohydrates for energy
RIBOFLAVIN (B2) RDA: 1.7 MG	Brewer's yeast, liver, milk, cheese, leafy green vegetables, enriched flour	For healthy skin, eyes, mucous membranes; helps body use protein, carbohydrates and fat for energy
NIACIN RDA: 20 MG	Brewer's yeast, peanut butter, meat, whole grain and enriched breads and cereals	For healthy skin and nerves; helps cells use oxygen to release energy

Major Nutrients, Their Sources, and Functions *(continued)*

Nutrient and Safe/Recom- mended Intake	Important Sources	Functions in the Human Body
PYRIDOXINE (B6) RDA: 2.0 MG	Meat, liver, whole grain cereals and breads, bananas, spinach, fish	For protein and fat metabolism; for red blood cell formation
FOLIC ACID RDA: 400 MCG	Broccoli and leafy green vegetables, liver, asparagus, lettuce, legumes	Aids in development of red blood cells
VITAMIN C RDA: 60 MG	Citrus fruit, berries, tomatoes, potatoes, chilis, peppers, leafy green vegetables, broccoli, lettuce	For healthy skin, gums, teeth, blood vessels; for wound healing and bone growth; helps use iron; helps resist infection
ZINC RDA: 15 MG	Liver, shellfish, brewer's yeast, wheat germ, eggs, whole grains	For wound healing; involved in normal growth and development
IRON RDA: 15 MG	Liver, red meat, shellfish, leafy green vegetables, whole grain and enriched cereal products, legumes	In red blood cells, iron carries oxygen to cells; for good immune and nerve functioning
CALCIUM RDA: 1000 MG	Milk, cheese, yogurt, leafy green vegetables, shellfish, sardines	For strong bones and teeth; aids in normal functioning of muscles, nerves, enzymes; aids in blood clotting

7

Coping with Hair Loss and Skin Changes

Most of the temporary changes caused by the side effects of chemotherapy happen inside your body. They aren't obvious to others. You cannot see a low white count or changes in appetite or digestion. But changes in your hair and skin happen outside your body and are visible. For many people, chemotherapy's effect on hair is especially difficult. The way you wear your hair is one of the ways you express your identity and individual style. Dealing with hair loss or hair thinning can be a hard, even traumatic, adjustment. Even though these changes are temporary, you still have to deal with them during the months of your treatment.

Not all chemotherapy medicines cause hair loss or skin changes. Your doctor or nurse will tell you about the specific chemotherapy drugs you are getting and any changes in your hair and skin that you might anticipate. As with the other potential side effects from chemotherapy, if you know what to expect, you'll be able to prepare and better cope with the problems.

This chapter will explain how chemotherapy can affect your hair and skin and what you can do to look good and feel good during this time.

How Does Chemotherapy Affect Hair?

Chemotherapy works by damaging cells that are rapidly dividing. As a result, cancer cells, which divide with great frequency, are extremely vulnerable to the effects of chemotherapy. But other cells which are dividing quickly can also be temporarily damaged.

Hair grows from follicles, which contain special cells that divide frequently to make your hair grow. Since at any one time about 90 percent of your hair follicles are in the active growth phase, they are especially susceptible to the effects of chemotherapy.

Hair loss occurs when chemotherapy drugs damage dividing follicle cells, producing weak, brittle hair that may break off at the scalp or fall out at the root itself. It is not just the hair on your head that may be affected. Some people notice that their eyebrows become thinner. But in general, since the hair on the rest of your body is not growing as rapidly as the hair on your head, you may not notice significant hair loss from other areas.

Will It Happen to Me?

Whether or not you lose your hair depends on the type and dosage of the chemotherapy drugs you receive. Some drugs may not affect your hair at all. Some may cause partial hair loss seen as hair thinning. And some chemotherapy drugs will cause complete hair loss. Your doctor or nurse will tell you what to expect from the specific drugs and dosages you are getting.

Is There Any Way To Prevent Hair Damage?

Chemotherapy is carried by the blood to the cells and then in a few hours is eliminated. If blood flow to the hair follicles can be reduced for a short time while the concentration of chemotherapy is highest, then the follicles would be less affected. People have tried various ways to temporarily reduce the blood flow to the scalp while getting chemotherapy.

One method uses a tight band around the scalp to reduce blood flow to the hair follicles while chemotherapy is going into the veins. The band is applied around your hairline before the chemotherapy is given and removed afterwards. Another method uses a special ice cap which chills the scalp and thus slows the blood flow to that area. The ice cap is applied for about a half hour before the chemotherapy goes in and stays on for about a half hour afterwards. If you use an ice cap, you may be more comfortable on a recliner or a bed rather than in a straight chair, because the cap can feel heavy. You may also want to ask your nurse for a warm blanket so that you don't feel chilled while wearing the ice cap.

Are These Methods Effective To Stop Hair Loss?

These methods of protecting the hair follicles from the effects of chemotherapy are limited. Certain drugs given in large doses will cause complete hair loss no matter what you do. These methods can only be used if chemotherapy is given over a relatively short period of time—over half an hour or so. If you receive the chemotherapy over several days while in the hospital, then using an ice cap or tight band on your scalp simply won't be possible.

In addition, there is some concern that preventing the chemotherapy from reaching your scalp will enable some cancer cells to escape the therapy. Ask your doctor how he or she feels about these methods of protecting your hair follicles and whether they are recommended for you.

When Will Hair Loss Happen?

Although damage to the hair follicle is immediate, you won't see the result of that damage until about a week or two later. Your scalp may feel very sensitive at first, and then you'll notice unusually large amounts of hair coming out on your brush or hair in the shower drain or on your pillow.

As more hair shafts break and less hair grows in because of the damage to the hair follicles, the remaining hair on your head will appear thinner. In some cases, hair loss will show up in patches.

When Will My Hair Grow Back?

Just like the cells of your digestive system or bone marrow, damaged hair follicles recover quickly. They start producing hair again right away. However, because the hair grows slowly, you probably won't notice hair growth before your next chemotherapy treatment, when the cycle is repeated. People who receive chemotherapy treatments every three or four weeks usually won't see hair growth begin to return until about a month or two after all chemotherapy treatments are completed.

When your hair returns, it will feel at first like "peach fuzz." Later you may notice a difference in texture. If your hair was curly before, the new hair may grow in straighter. Previously straight hair may grow in curly. Your hair may be finer or coarser than it was before, your hair may grow in darker or lighter than your natural color. But if your hair grows back differently at first, over time it may return to its original color and texture.

Coping with Hair Loss

Even when people expect to lose their hair from chemotherapy, it's still upsetting when it actually happens. Since there is a delay of about a week or so from the chemotherapy treatment to when the hair loss actually starts, you may be long gone from the hospital or clinic. And you may not have the support of nurses or other medical staff who are familiar with what is happening to you. This is a good time to get involved in a cancer support group where you'll find others who have faced these same problems (see Chapter 10 for more information). Don't hesitate to check back in with the advice nurse at your oncologist's office. And remind yourself that *this is temporary*, and that *your hair will return* when your chemotherapy treatments are over.

Many people find it distressing to see their hair clogging the drain or filling their brush. If your hair is long, it may be helpful to have your hair cut into a shorter style before starting chemotherapy treatments that cause hair loss.

About Wigs

If you plan to get a wig, it will be helpful to take some photographs of your hairline and your hair style from the front, side, and back. Also snip little samples of your hair from the front and back as well. This will enable you to match the wig's color and style to your own hair.

Purchase your wig from a store which can provide experienced sales staff, privacy, and individual attention. If you are unsure about where to go, ask your nurse or the American Cancer Society for a referral.

There are a number of things to consider when buying a wig, in order to make it as natural looking and comfortable as possible.

Type of Wig. Wigs can be made of different materials. A synthetic fiber wig is less expensive, but tends to be stiff. It must be dry cleaned instead of shampooed and cannot be styled with a curling iron or permanent. Although Asian or European hair is more expensive, it looks more natural and can be washed as well as styled. Asian hair will be coarser and straighter than European hair.

Wig construction. The way a wig is constructed affects its comfort and how natural it looks. If the wig has a mesh base, it must be dry cleaned and cannot take a perm. More expensive "customized" wigs have hair that is implanted into a "skin" base and are more comfortable.

Fit. It is very important that the wig fits you well. If you are constantly aware of the wig, if you are afraid to move in a natural way because it is uncomfortable, then you won't feel good wearing it. The wig isn't serving its purpose. Buying a wig while you still have some hair can be a problem because it may not fit as well after all your hair is gone. Be sure to have the wig refitted, if necessary, to assure comfort.

How you attach a wig can make a big difference. One way a wig can be attached to your head is with small pieces of a special kind of tape. The tape attaches to your hairline and the base of the wig. Whatever way the wig is attached, it should feel secure. You should be able to move your head and bend over without worrying that the wig will slip.

Comfort. Your body generates heat, and when you perspire the air evaporates the moisture and cools you down. You might not normally notice the perspiration from your head, but it can be a problem when you wear a wig. The air isn't able to reach your scalp, and you may notice the perspiration making your scalp itch or feel hot. This can make wearing your wig uncomfortable. To overcome the problem, try wrapping a thin cotton scarf around your head under the wig. Or you can get a piece of stretchy stockinette material that can be tied at one end to make a cap. This can then be worn under the wig, and it will help absorb perspiration as well as provide a cushion between your wig and your scalp.

Cost. The price of wigs can vary from $50 to several thousand dollars. The cost may be covered by insurance if the doctor writes you a "prescription" for a "wig prosthesis." Prosthesis is the medical term for "replacement of a missing part by an artificial substitute." Most physicians are aware of the wording required when petitioning the insurance company to reimburse you for the cost of your wig. Be sure to remind your doctor that the prescription must also indicate the *medical necessity* for the wig (for example, "Alopecia (hair loss) due to chemotherapy"). If your insurance can offset some of the cost of the wig, you may be able to afford a more expensive and natural looking one.

Alternatives to Wigs

Many women use scarves and head wraps as alternatives to wearing a wig. It is a way to add color, texture, and accents to their wardrobe. A basic cotton square folded into two uneven triangles and tied at the back of your neck can be both colorful and comfortable. You can add a contrasting color by twisting another scarf into a cord and tying that around the first scarf. You can also experiment with side knots or adding a hat or a beret over the scarf.

While at home or at night you might try a soft terry cotton turban. It's an easy and comfortable alternative to a wig or head wrap. The American Cancer Society often provides turbans, free of charge, to people receiving chemotherapy. Baseball caps have also proven popular with both men and women. They're colorful and can be worn either with or without a head wrap.

If you choose not to use any head covering, you need to be aware of the weather. Hair serves as an insulation and protects your body from losing heat. In colder weather you'll need a hat or scarf. Your hair also protects your scalp prom the ultraviolet rays of the sun, so you'll need a hat or sunscreen (at least SP 15) while you are in direct sunlight.

How To Cope with Thinning Hair

As previously noted, not all chemotherapy medicines cause complete hair loss. But they may cause your hair to become dry, brittle, and thinner than usual. Because your hair is more fragile, you should be especially gentle in your hair care. Wash and dry your hair gently—it's even more fragile wet than when it's dry. Check with your barber or hairdresser for special products made to be used with "overtreated" or "damaged" hair. Avoid harsh chemicals like peroxide or permanents. And don't use a hot blow dryer or hot curlers. They'll make your hair even dryer and more likely to break.

Many people find that shorter hair camouflages the problem of thinning. Longer hair is heavier, and the weight pulls it flatter on your head. Hair which is shorter tends to spring upwards and contributes to a fuller look.

If your hair is very long, you may want to cut it a little at a time. The change won't be so drastic, and you'll have the chance to gradually adjust to a different look.

Don't forget the importance of eating a well-balanced diet to keep your hair healthy. Poor nutrition due to nausea or a diminished appetite may contribute to your hair looking dull and lifeless. Chapter 6 contains suggestions about how to maintain a balanced diet while getting chemotherapy.

Skin and Nails

Dryness

Dry skin can be caused by a number of different factors— the effects of chemotherapy, antinausea medication, dehydration, or poor nutrition. Skin can also be dry and sensitive from the effects of radiation. Dry skin is not only uncomfortable and sometimes itchy, but it's also more likely to be damaged by normal activities. Here are some general suggestions to prevent and treat dry, itchy skin.

- Lubricate your skin after washing with a water-based moisturizer.

- Take warm rather than hot baths or showers, because hot water can actually dry skin.

- Use a moisturizing soap such as Aveno, which can save your skin from the overdrying effects of regular soap.

- Avoid alcohol-based products, because they have the effect of drying your skin.

- Avoid letting wool or other scratchy fabrics come in contact with your skin.

- Soft, loose cotton clothing is less irritating than tight-fitting clothing that may bind or cause more irritation to skin that is already dry.

Sunburn

Some chemotherapy drugs will make your skin more sensitive to the sun. This means that sun exposure that would ordinarily not affect you could cause a burn. If the chemotherapy drugs you receive cause increased sun sensitivity, take precautions. Use sunscreen with a sun protection level of at least SP 15. (SP 15 means you can be in the sun fifteen times longer than you normally can without burning.) Be generous with sunscreen to specially vulnerable areas of your skin. Using lip gloss with sunscreen will protect your lips. Wear a hat with a wide enough brim to protect your face and long sleeves and long pants to protect your arms and legs. Remember that even on hazy days the sun's rays can penetrate to cause a burn.

Tanning

The color of your skin is the result of the amount of melanin it contains. Dark-skinned people have more melanin than light-skinned people. Your pituitary gland produces a melanin-stimulating hormone (MSH) that determines your complexion. When you are exposed to the sun, your pituitary is stimulated to produce more melanin, thus bringing about the normal tanning process. Some chemotherapy drugs stimulate your body to make more melanin than usual, and as a result your skin may become darker temporarily. This may be noticeable in your nailbeds (the skin under your nails), on the skin over your joints, or in the mucous membranes of your mouth.

If you're getting chemotherapy through an IV into the veins of your hands or arms, you may develop a darkening in the skin over your veins. It may seem that the patterns of the veins in your hands or arms are outlined in a color several shades darker than your normal skin tone. (If you are getting chemotherapy into larger veins near your heart through an implanted port or central catheter, you won't see this darkening pattern.) Sometimes the darkening effect is evenly distributed over your body, like a regular suntan. People with darker skin may be more likely to develop the darkening effect than people with lighter skin.

Skin reaction, whatever its extent, is temporary. You may notice it beginning two to three weeks after the start of chemotherapy, and it will start to fade away after your treatment is completed.

Your skin may become temporarily flushed looking for a few days after receiving the chemotherapy drug Etoposide. Most of the time the flushing will occur in a localized area, especially on your face or neck. The flushing is not painful, although the redness can be fairly bright. Unlike the tanning effect, which can last for a long time, the flushing will usually disappear a few days after your treatment.

Radiation Recall

If you are receiving chemotherapy at the same time or very shortly after getting radiation therapy, you may develop a skin condition called *radiation recall*. Radiation recall appears as redness or dry peeling of skin that has been radiated. This may be caused by the effect of the chemotherapy interfering with the repair of skin cells damaged by radiation. If this happens, you should consult with the doctor and the nurses in the radiation department for their suggestions about special skin care. They may suggest washing the area with mild soap and drying it gently or avoiding irritating clothes, exposure to the sun, and extremes in heat (heating pads, hot water bottles, hot showers) or cold (ice packs or cold wind). They may also prescribe an ointment to promote healing. .

Allergic Reactions

At any time—not just during chemotherapy—you can have an allergic skin reaction to a particular medicine. An allergic skin reaction may appear as raised, red, or itchy bumps on your skin. If this happens, you should check with your doctor or nurses as soon as possible. They will likely prescribe medication, such as an antihistamine or steroid, to stop the allergic reaction. The itchiness of an allergic skin reaction can be quite irritating, and an untreated reaction may cause other skin problems or infections.

Changes in Your Nails

Your nails grow from under the skin at the base of your cuticle. Chemotherapy's effect on these growing cells can cause your nails to be brittle and grow at a slower rate than usual. After several weeks, when the part of your nail that was under your cuticle when you received chemotherapy grows out to where it's visible, you may see a white band or ridge in the nail. As your nail continues to grow and the white band moves closer to the tip of your finger, you may find that the nail may break more easily, peel, or catch on your clothing.

To prevent your nails from tearing, you should clip them close to your fingertips. Some people find that tape or bandaids effectively prevent snagging while that fragile band or ridge grows out. Your nails are the best protection against pain or infection in the nail beds, so try to let the ridges grow out naturally, without peeling them off early and exposing the nail bed to damage.

You should not use artificial nails at this time. Nor should you use alcohol-based polish or polish remover, as these will only add to the problem of breaking and peeling. Any nail polish remover you use should be lanolin-based.

Looking Good

Appearance and body image are important to nearly everyone. You need to have effective ways to cope with the temporary changes in your appearance caused by chemotherapy. A number of resources offer solid help so that you can look better and feel better about yourself. The American Cancer Society has put together a program called "Look Good ... Feel Better." It's taught by specially trained cosmetologists who help people who are dealing with changes in their appearance due to chemotherapy. Their classes offer tips on how you can apply makeup, use scarves creatively, and camouflage skin change. Ask your nurse or call the American Cancer Society to see if there is a class available near you.

The book *Beauty and Cancer*, by Dianne Doan Noyes and Peggy Mellody, (L. S. Press, 1988), has many ideas for hair care, wigs, makeup, nutrition, and exercise. The authors also provide the names of beauty supplies, beauty consultants, and support agencies that specialize in hair and beauty care for your special needs while getting chemotherapy.

8

Sexuality and Fertility

Any health problem can strongly affect your emotions. When you are coping with cancer and the stress of cancer-fighting treatments, you can feel overwhelmed. You may be worried or even angry about your diagnosis. You may feel pressured by the decisions you are being asked to make about your treatment or be fearful about your ability to survive. If you are recovering from recent surgery, you may still feel some pain and exhaustion. You may be adjusting to changes in your body from the illness or from surgery. If you have lost a part of your body (visible or not), you may still be grieving.

If you are in a relationship, your partner can be going through many of these same feelings—worry, depression, anger, and grief. These stresses can disrupt the balance of the relationship. Your need for contact, acceptance, and physical comfort may be even greater now, yet your partner may hold back. He or she may feel overwhelmed or hesitate to initiate physical contact for fear of harming you or adding to your stress.

If sexual contact was something you valued and enjoyed before your illness, your *feelings* probably haven't changed. But now you may have questions about how the illness or its treatments may affect your *ability* to be sexual. You may not feel comfortable asking your doctor or nurse about these concerns: questions about sex may seem unimportant or inappropriate in comparison to the "life and death" issues that they are dealing with. But information about how cancer or cancer treatments affect you sexually is important to your recovery. When is it safe to resume sexual intercourse? How will the medicine you are taking affect you sexually? Will you still be able to have an erection or experience orgasm?

Many myths about sex and cancer cause people much unnecessary anguish. Your mother may have complained that she was no longer interested in sex after her hysterectomy. Is that going to be true for you as well? You may worry that sexual activity may be harmful or painful after surgery, especially if the surgery involved the reproductive organs or breasts. You may worry that the cancer was caused by sexual activity. Some people fear that they can give cancer to their partner by intimate contact.

These myths are not only untrue, but also damaging. If either you or your partner fall under the influence of unfounded notions like these, you can end up cutting each other off from the nourshing enjoyment of a sexual relationship.

One way of dispelling a myth is to ask your doctor or nurse about your concerns and get the facts clarified. If you do ask, you will learn that hormonal changes, menopausal symptoms, hysterectomy, or breast surgery do not necessarily mean the end of sexual enjoyment. Prostate or bowel surgery doesn't necessarily mean that a man can no longer have an erection or experience orgasm. Sex is not harmful to the person recovering from cancer, nor will it spread the disease.

The following sections will help you understand some of the basic facts regarding cancer and sexuality.

Sensation and Circulation

All sensations, whether or not they are sexual, depend on the nerves carrying information to and from your brain via the spinal cord. Nerves to the sexual organs can be damaged from the pressure of a tumor on the nerves, the spinal cord, or the brain. These nerves can also be damaged as a result of the surgery done to remove the cancer. Fortunately, today's improved surgical techniques are less damaging to the organs, nerves, and blood supply that affect sexual functioning. Medications can also affect your nerves. Some chemotherapy medicines can cause numbness in your fingers, which will change how you experience certain kinds of sensation. Other medicines that you may be taking to relieve pain or nausea can also diminish sexual responsiveness.

Hormonal Changes

A hormone is a chemical substance produced by one organ that is carried by the blood and so affects other organs. For instance, insulin is a hormone produced by your pancreas. It is carried by the blood to other cells in your body and allows them to absorb or use sugar. Other hormones affect the rate of metabolism (thyroxine, produced by the thyroid gland) or rate of growth (somatotropin, also called growth hormone, produced by the pituitary gland).

The sex hormones are responsible for the development of secondary sex characteristics and fertility in both men and women. These hormones are produced in the mature reproductive organs (ovaries in women, testes in men). Small amounts of both estrogen and testosterone are also produced in the adrenal glands, located near the kidneys. Although both sexes produce estrogen (the female sex homrone) and testosterone (the male sex hormone), men produce a great deal more of testosterone, and women produce a great deal more of estrogen.

At puberty, testosterone causes the male genitals to enlarge and the testes to produce sperm. It also stimulates the development of other characteristics, such as male distribution of body hair, voice changes, body build, and sex drive. Although the level of testosterone may slow down as a man ages, a man can continue to produce testosterone and sperm for his entire life.

In women, estrogen is responsible for the increase in size of the reproductive organs (uterus, cervix, vagina, ovaries), female distribution of body hair, body build, and the development of breasts. Since most of a woman's estrogen is produced in the ovaries, when these secretions slow down during menopause, the drop in the estrogen level causes a number of physical changes. Without estrogen, the vaginal lining is thinner, drier, and less elastic. The supply of blood to the vagina also decreases. The cervix (the bottom of the uterus) produces less mucous, and less lubrication is produced during sexual arousal.

The hormonal changes of menopause normally happen slowly over a number of years. But if the ovaries have been removed by surgery or stop functioning because of medications or the effects of chemotherapy, a sudden drop in estrogen can result. This decrease in estrogen will cause changes in the vaginal lining and secretions. Characteristic "hot flashes" can be more frequent and severe than with normal menopause. Some women can take hormone pills which replace estrogen (as well as other hormones) and relieve many menopausal symptoms. But some kinds of cancer can also be stimulated to grow more rapidly in the presence of estrogen, so hormone replacement therapy (HRT) is not recommended for everyone.

Men can also be affected by hormonal changes. If surgery, medication, or chemotherapy reduces the production of testosterone, a man may experience some loss of sexual drive. Over time he will notice changes in hair distribution as well as changes in muscle and fat distribution. As with women, some cancers in men grow more rapidly in the presence of sex hormones, and in these cases doctors may prescribe antiandrogen hormones to turn off testosterone production. Some new, nonsteriod antiandrogens are effective in lowering testosterone levels while having less detrimental effects on a man's sexual drive or ability to have an erection.

If a man loses his ability to maintain an erection because of surgery, reduced testosterone levels, or drugs, there are several options to consider. When the organic causes can't be corrected or reversed, some men choose to have a penile implant. One type of implant is a semi-rigid penile rod that keeps the penis partially erect at all times. A second option is a prosthesis that uses self-controlled inflatable rods. This type of implant inflates or deflates via manual manipulation of the penis. Instead of a prosthesis, some men prefer changing their sexual behavior to focus more on oral sex and manual touching for giving and receiving pleasure. This option has worked for many couples.

Changes in Body Image

Your body image is the picture you have in your mind about your physical self. That picture helps form a sense of who you are. A positive body image allows you to feel whole, acceptable, and lovable. When that picture changes, there is necessarily a period of adjustment until you can adapt to the new sense of who you are.

People react very differently to physical changes. Some women experience a hysterectomy as a relief. They are rid of their menstrual periods and no longer have to worry about birth control. Other women may grieve for the loss of their uterus and menstrual periods because this loss signifies the end of the potential for having children and the disappearance of a function that is tied to their femininity and sexuality. Even if their uterus contained cancer cells and the surgery to remove it may have been life-saving, the hysterectomy can still be felt as a loss and a change in body image that takes time to integrate.

Just having cancer can be tremendously disturbing to your body image, especially if you've always felt strong and healthy. Surgery or other treatments that alter your body either temporarily or permanently can be even more traumatic, and when these changes are noticeable and disfiguring, the natural process of grieving lasts longer. It can profoundly affect your self-esteem, confidence, and sexuality. If you dread looking at your scar after breast surgery or at your stoma after bowel surgery, you are likely to worry about how your partner will react or how these changes will affect the way you share your body during intimate sexual contact.

The effects of chemotherapy can greatly alter your body image as well. Hair loss is perhaps the greatest assault to your picture of yourself, but pallor and weight changes can also make you feel self-conscious about your body. A temporary intravenous line that emerges from your chest may feel foreign and obtrusive. Fatigue, nausea, or the sedating effects of pain and antinausea medication can prevent you from feeling sexual in your usual way. Your body may not feel like it belongs to you anymore, but to the doctors and nurses. It is no wonder that many people are reluctant to reestablish sexual contact while feeling this way.

Adjusting to Body Image Changes

The way you react to the physical changes caused by cancer and anticancer treatments is personal. The amount of time it takes to adjust to these changes varies from person to person and from couple to couple. There is no right timetable, nor is there an ideal way that couples should deal with these problems. Some people are comfortable sharing the entire experience with their partner, having him or her present during doctors' visits, dressing changes, and any educational or supportive contact they have with other health-care professionals. In that way, they learn together and are able to reinforce the information for each other. Partners can ask their own questions and be advocates. Other people want more independence, preferring to absorb the information at their own pace and share the information with their partner as they are able.

For some people, reconstructive surgery makes a big difference in how they feel about their body; all the physical adjustments seem easier. Other people feel that the additional surgery would be traumatic, especially at a time when they may still be facing months of chemotherapy. Reconstruction would be something they'd consider after treatment is over, if at all. In any case, feeling whole and attractive and sexual is *not* dependent on reconstructive surgery. A number of studies comparing women who have had breast-conserving surgery (lumpectomy with radiation therapy) to women who have had a mastectomy (surgical removal of the entire breast) do show that women who have had breast-conserving surgery feel less self-conscious about their bodies (especially when nude). But there is *no* significant difference in their psychological distress, marital happiness, frequency of sex, or level of sexual satisfaction (Dr. Leslie Schover, (March/April 1991) "The Impact of Breast Cancer on Sexuality, Body Image, and Intimate Relationships," *Ca-A Journal for Clinicians.* Vol. 41,2:112-119.)

Some people are more comfortable if they camouflage changes in their body when they are intimate. There are soft, fiber-filled "night" bras that can be worn under nightgowns to camouflage a missing breast. To cover a stoma and collection bag, some women will wear a "teddy" or T-shirt to bed, or men can wear a soft cotton cummerbund. Other couples feel closer to their partners if they can share themselves as freely as they did before their surgery and grow used to the changes together over time. Either choice is fine; it's a matter of doing what feels comfortable for you.

Dealing with Pain and Discomfort

Even though the doctor assures you that it's physically safe to resume sexual relations, you may not feel ready. You may need more time to heal, physically and emotionally. Or you may want to engage only in gentle sex play or sex that doesn't involve intercourse. Good communication is more important now than ever if you are to find a way to share sexual intimacy that is satisfying to both of you. Go slow. Let your partner know how you're feeling and what is comfortable for you. Your partner may be so fearful of harming you that he or she is reluctant to initiate sexual activity at all, and your encouragement and assurance is important.

If you take pain medication or a muscle relaxer, be sure to allow at least a half hour for it to work. Be aware that medications can also make you sleepy or limit your arousal. A warm bath or soothing massage is another way to feel more comfortable before sex.

You may find that certain positions are more comfortable for you or that you need to use a pillow to protect a tender incision or support a part of your body for comfort. Let yourself experiment with ways of pleasuring each other that allow you to feel close without pushing your physical or emotional limits.

For women, the lack of estrogen can make intercourse painful because of the changes in their vaginal lining and lack of natural lubrication. If intercourse causes irritation, use a water-based lubricant or a vaginal suppository. Some women can use an estrogen cream to counteract the effects of menopause on their vaginal tissue.

Fertility

Many couples who hope to have children in the future are concerned about how cancer or the cancer-fighting treatments will affect their fertility. This is an important issue to discuss with your doctor. Whether or not it is possible to preserve reproductive functioning depends on a number of things—the kind of cancer you have and your sex and age, as well as the amount, duration, and type of chemotherapy medicines and radiation you receive. In general, every attempt will be made to preserve your fertility without jeopardizing the effectiveness of your treatment. For some people, the effects on fertility will not be known for sure until after all the treatments are over and their body has a chance to return to normal.

Men. The layer of the testes that produces sperm is constantly dividing. Since chemotherapy has the strongest effect on the cells that are frequently dividing, it can have a more detrimental effect on a man's production of sperm than a woman's monthly maturation of a single ovum (egg). When a man receives chemotherapy, his sperm production can decrease or stop altogether. And the sperm that is produced will have less motility, so that they are less able to reach the ovum to fertilize it.

Some chemotherapy medicines are more damaging to fertility than others. If protecting fertility is an important issue, it may be possible to substitute a different drug that will be less damaging to the sperm-producing cells of the testes. As a general rule for chemotherapy, the larger the dose and the longer the period of treatment, the more likely it is that your fertility will be affected.

If it is possible that your treatment may cause infertility, you can consider preserving your sperm in a sperm bank. The sperm is kept frozen for an indefinite period of time. When you want to have a child, the sperm can be thawed and used for artificial insemination of your partner. Preserving your sperm may *not* be possible if the cancer has caused abnormal sperm or decreased sperm motility. If you are interested in preserving your sperm, ask your doctor or nurse to refer you to a sperm bank in your area where the process is handled in a professional manner, with sensitivity to your feelings and need for privacy.

Women. Even though the ovum-producing layer of the ovary is less damaged by chemotherapy, a woman's fertility is still at risk. Chemotherapy often causes menstrual periods to stop during treatment. For older women, closer to the end of their childbearing years, the periods may not return, resulting in a premature menopause. As with men, the kind of chemotherapy, dose, and length of treatment are all factors which will influence whether the ovary will continue to produce mature eggs and secrete the hormones necessary for conception.

Women who are facing potential loss of fertility may want to save their eggs or embryos (fertilized eggs) for the future. This process is not as simple as sperm banking. It requires much more time, hormonal stimulation to produce multiple eggs, and more medical intervention. All three of these factors can delay your chemotherapy treatment and recovery. Ask your doctor if you can safely consider this alternative.

Both men and women should continue to use effective birth control during treatment because chemotherapy can damage the sperm or the embryo.

Protecting Your Sexuality

If a surgery or medication will cause changes in your ability to function sexually, even temporarily, you need to know about it ahead of time. Physicians (especially surgeons) recognize their obligation to provide you with enough information so you understand the reason, risks, and alternatives to their recommended treatment. If your regular visits to the oncology office or clinic are too brief to allow you to discuss your concerns, you and your partner can make a "talking" appointment with your physician. Plan a list of questions important to you. How will your ability to enjoy sex be affected? Will it affect your sexual desire? Your ability to have an erection or orgasm? Does the doctor expect that the problem will be temporary, reversible, or permanent? When will you and your partner be able to resume your normal sexual activities?

If your physician can't answer your questions, he or she may refer you to a specialist for further evaluation. A urologist is a specialist in the urinary tract of both sexes and the genital and reproductive functioning of men. A neurologist is a specialist in diseases involving the nerves and sensation of your body, including the brain and spinal cord. A vascular specialist will evaluate how your blood supply to different organs can be affected by surgery, medication, or the cancer itself.

In some cases, short-term sexual counseling with your partner can give both of you the opportunity to explore feelings, fears, and needs around sexuality. A specialist may also be a resource for learning about other positions or means of stimulation that will maximize your enjoyment during this time. Support groups can also be helpful, especially if the group includes others who have had the same kind of cancer or the same kind of cancer-fighting treatment. You may get some ideas about how other couples are dealing with the changes in their sexual lives.

Coping

Your sexuality is not located in any specific organ, nor is it limited to any specific activity. It's much more than that. Your sexuality is a refletion of how you feel about yourself as a man or a woman. It depends in part on your acceptance and appreciation of your body as a source of pleasure to you and your partner. Your sexuality is shaped by your memories and experiences, and it changes all through your life. Your illness may change to some degree how you express your sexuality, but it won't change your need to give and receive some form of loving sexual touch.

Your ability to establish and maintain a sexual connection with someone contributes to the quality of your life. Even though in times of stress or illnesses "having sex" may be the last thing on your mind, the need to love and care for another and to be loved and cared for in return is always there. Sexual contact is something that is not only possible during your illness and treatments; it can be a source of comfort, reassurance, passion, and joy.

9

Coping with Fatigue

In our society, it is not uncommon to hear people complaining about feeling tired and worn out. The stresses of living in a highly technical and constantly changing world contribute to this sensation of fatigue. But for a person facing cancer and its treatments, fatigue can take on a new meaning. Many factors contribute to this problem—the physical and psychological toll of the disease and the effects of chemotherapy, radiation, or other medications. This chapter will focus on some of the causes of fatigue in a person receiving chemotherapy and provide suggestions for managing them so that you feel better.

Why Does It Happen?

Physical Causes

There are obvious physical reasons for feeling tired. Before people are diagnosed with cancer, one of the first symptoms they may notice is generalized fatigue. Depending upon the location and type of cancer, it may be affecting the normal processes of the body. If the cancer is in the bone marrow, the body is unable to make enough red blood cells to carry needed oxygen to each of the body's cells. If the cancer is affecting other organs, your body may be unable to fully metabolize waste or absorb needed nutrients. Anything that interrupts your body's normal functioning is likely to make you tired.

As you have read, cancer cells reproduce more rapidly than normal cells. This rapid reproduction leads other cells to break down as well. When cells die or are destroyed, they release the substances they carry inside themselves. An increased amount of these substances can tax the normal function of your body and cause you to feel tired.

Pain can be yet another reason for fatigue. Not all cancers are painful, but if you have aches and pains related to the disease, dealing with these can be very tiring. Many people are able to minimize the pain they feel by using distraction or "just not thinking about it." Unfortunately, this also takes a lot of energy to accomplish. Pain is often more noticeable at night and can prevent people from sleeping well. Even if you spend eight hours in bed at night, your sleep may not be as restful when you are having pain.

In addition to oxygen to help the body's cells to work, every body needs nutrients. Any upset of the stomach and intestines (such as nausea, vomiting, diarrhea, or constipation) can disturb your ability to eat and rob you of your energy.

Fevers due to the cancer or to infections related to a weakened immune system can also leave you feeling weak and tired. An increase in body temperature not only makes cells work harder, but also leads them to need more oxygen and nutrients to perform their jobs.

Stress

Stress is another major source of fatigue. Most likely, your life did not revolve around going to the doctor or the hospital before your diagnosis. Once you have been diagnosed, you may need to juggle your schedule to fit in all the appointments you will have. If you are also trying to keep up with other responsibilities, such as work or caring for your family, this added stress may contribute significantly to your feeling of fatigue.

Treatment-Related Causes

Besides the physical reasons for fatigue, people with cancer often feel tired because of the treatments themselves. If you have had major surgery to remove the cancer, you may be very tired from the procedure. If you had general anesthesia during the surgery, its effects may take some time to wear off. The medicines used to control surgical pain can also cause you to be drowsy and tired. And the pain from the surgery may keep you from sleeping well.

Being in the hospital after surgery can also contribute to a sense of weariness. It is often difficult to sleep in the hospital, because it is an unfamiliar environment. Your normal bedtime routine, which helps you to relax into sleep, is disrupted. You may also experience frequent interruptions of your sleep from hospital staff performing various observations and tasks. The machines used in the hospital to help with your care make noises, too.

If you are taking chemotherapy as part of your treatment, side effects from these treatments can contribute to fatigue. While not all drugs cause this problem, one of the most common side effects of chemotherapy is the effect of the drugs on your bone marrow. If you become anemic because your bone marrow cannot produce enough red blood cells, this decrease will diminish the number of available red blood cells needed to carry oxygen to the other cells of your body. With less oxygen available to your cells, they are unable to perform their functions as they normally would. The effects of this process will be weakness and a feeling of fatigue.

Fortunately, treatment-related anemia is usually short in duration. If you are very anemic, your physician may decide to give you a transfusion of red blood cells. The transfused cells supplement the oxygen-carrying capacity of your own cells until your bone marrow recovers. Many people say that they feel more energetic after they have received a transfusion of red cells. Your doctor will explain the risks and benefits of this treatment for anemia.

Anemia can also be caused by a lack of a hormone (erythropoietin) that stimulates red blood cells to mature. An injection of a synthetic form of this hormone may increase the number of mature red blood cells and improve the anemia.

Another cause of fatigue directly related to chemotherapy is the effect of the cancer cells being destroyed. As cancer cells die, they create waste products that the kidneys and liver must manage. These waste products can tax your other organs and cause you to feel more tired.

Many people complain of feeling tired during their radiation treatments. The fatigue which comes from radiation does not occur suddenly, but rather over time. People describe it as a cumulative effect. Just as with chemotherapy, radiation therapy can also affect your bone marrow. Juggling your previous commitments to fit in daily radiation treatments may also increase your stress level and create more "work" for you.

A form of therapy used to treat cancer called *biological response modifiers* can also contribute to fatigue. Medications like interferon or interleukin-2 either help your own immune system combat the cancer or act like naturally occurring substances in your body which fight diseases. Unfortunately, some common side effects of these treatments are a flu-like syndrome and fatigue. If you are taking one of these drugs, you are likely to feel generally "blah" or suffer from a sense of malaise during the course of treatment.

If you experience other side effects from your treatments, these may also be the cause for fatigue. Nausea and vomiting can be very taxing. A sense of low-level queasiness or "just not feeling good" can be tiring too. In addition, medications used to treat the side effects of therapy can add to your feeling of being tired. Antinausea drugs such as Compazine or Ativan can be sedating. Decadron is a steroid drug used in treating nausea which can make people feel "wired" or more awake. During the day, this feeling of being more alert can be okay, but at night you may have trouble falling asleep. Unfortunately, because of the medications used, many people have problems getting as much sleep as they need. They complain that they are "too tired" to sleep. This excessive tiredness means they cannot sleep after their treatments.

Psychological Factors

Among the most obvious reasons for feeling fatigued when you have been diagnosed with cancer are the psychological factors. Feelings of worry and anxiety are a normal response to a diagnosis of a life-threatening illness, and these feelings often lead to difficulty sleeping at night.

Your mind may race with questions. Why did this happen to you? Can it really be happening? After the initial shock of the diagnosis has passed, you may find yourself worrying about the future. How serious is it? What will the outcome be? What kinds of treatments are available? What are your options? If you have relatives or friends who have undergone previous cancer treatments or have heard stories about cancer therapies, you may ask yourself whether your experience will be similar, better, or worse.

You may have the additional concern of wondering how your family will manage. If you have children, just talking to them about your diagnosis may be painful or difficult. Economic concerns may be preying on your mind. If you provide support for your family, you may be concerned about how they will manage if you cannot work. Health insurance coverage or paying for the medical care are other financial worries. Your role in the family may be changing as well. While you are receiving treatment and dealing with your cancer, you may worry that you won't be able to function in your full capacity.

All of these very practical issues can create sleep disturbances. In addition, it is not uncommon to feel down or depressed. Although many books written today stress being "up" or positive when facing cancer, acknowledging how *you* feel is an important component of living. In light of the challenges people with cancer face, it is certainly not unusual to feel overwhelmed or out of control. Facing cancer may mean that you undergo periods of feeling unhappy or depressed. These feelings will come and go, alternating with more positive times. But during the moments when you are "down," you are also likely to feel more tired and fatigued.

The causes of fatigue as they relate to cancer can be multiple and varied. Fortunately, there are a number of things you can do to deal with fatigue.

Self-Help Suggestions

Depending upon the cause of your fatigue, a variety of treatments may be available, and you should certainly explore these possibilities with your doctor. The suggestions given here provide a number of additional strategies that you can try to help yourself manage this problem.

Communication

Recognition that fatigue is a common problem when dealing with cancer and its treatments is an important first step in coping with it. Communicate how you are feeling. If you enlist your friends and family members to help when you are tired, you will be able to conserve energy. Many people will be eager to lend a hand if only you ask.

It is okay to let people know you are tired and need to rest. Visitors are eager to offer support, but often forget that they are not the only ones to "drop by" for a few hours. After several groups of visitors have come to see you, you may be extremely weary. If your friends understand ahead of time that you want to see them but may be feeling tired and want to spend only a short time talking, misunderstandings can be prevented.

Pacing

Pace yourself. Just as a long-distance runner doesn't go all out in the beginning of the race and become too exhausted to finish, you have to pace yourself throughout the day. Try to do one or two of your errands and then rest for a short time. After your rest, perform one or two more tasks and rest again. Many of us want to finish everything on our lists before we take a break. In fact, we believe if we work this way, we will then be able to take a very long break after everything is finished. Unfortunately, by the time the long break comes around, you will be exhausted. If you are starting out feeling tired already, a marathon of errands will only lead to more fatigue. Listen to your body. Use your fatigue level as a gauge for taking breaks. And take the break when you are starting to feel tired. Don't push yourself till you have zero energy. If you have trouble listening to your body, simply schedule regular periods for rest during the day and follow your schedule.

Prioritize the chores you need to do, ranking them by their importance and the amount of energy that each task will take. Then schedule them in the order that will be least tiring. For example, if you have more energy in the morning, plan to do something that will take more time and energy early in the day. Save the lighter tasks for the late afternoon when you may be more tired.

Another pacing technique is to *avoid* taking long naps during the day. Disturbances in sleep cycles can occur after hospitalizations or from medications such as steroids. If you are sleeping for long periods during the day, you may find yourself sleeping either fitfully or not at all at night.

To correct a problem of altered sleeping patterns, try to reestablish your normal habits by going to bed at the usual time. By not sleeping for extended periods during the daytime, you will probably be tired enough to fall asleep when you retire. When you feel the need to rest during the day, try sitting quietly and relaxing by listening to soft music. Or just go into your room, close the door, and lie down for a few minutes.

Even if you don't nap for hours during the day, you still may find yourself struggling to fall asleep. Rather than tossing and turning in bed, go ahead and get up. Try drinking a warm glass of milk or an herbal tea like chamomile. Reading a light book can be helpful as well. Or try some of the relaxation suggestions below. It may take a little time to revert back to your usual sleep patterns, but, with a little help, you can do it.

Relaxation Techniques

If your fatigue is related to stress, anxiety, or an inability to sleep, relaxation and visualization techniques may be helpful. A very informal way to relax is to take ten minutes in the midst of a hectic day to sit in a quiet place by yourself without thinking about what needs to be done next. The old saying about "stopping to smell the roses" is appropriate when we feel stressed. Thinking about the beautiful rose or the warm sun takes our minds out of the whirling activity in which we often find ourselves. Don't worry that you don't have the time or that all the things that need to be done will keep intruding into your mind. You do have the time, and if the thoughts do intrude, that is okay.

More formal relaxation techniques are used by many people. A method called progressive muscle relaxation lets you systematically focus on and then relax groups of muscles. Full instructions for progressive muscle relaxation are covered in Chapter 11. A side benefit of relaxation techniques is that they can often lead to a period of sleep. You can find a script for relaxation and guided imagery in Chapter 12.

Counseling and Social Support

If your fatigue is caused by psychological factors, you might consider seeking professional counseling. A professional will be objective and nonjudgmental. Having someone like that to talk with about your worries and concerns can be very helpful. A counselor may also be able to help you find new ways to manage your concerns and stress.

Support groups for cancer patients are also helpful. Sometimes just talking to other cancer patients about their fatigue can be beneficial. It is often helpful to know you are not the only person to experience this sense of weariness. In addition, many people are happy to discuss ways they have worked out to assist them in dealing with stress or sleep problems. More on the ways that support groups might help you in dealing with problems encountered during chemotherapy use can be found in Chapter 10.

Dietary Techniques

Nutritional problems may be contributing to your sense of tiredness. You may be having difficulty eating enough food to provide the materials your body needs to make energy. Are you nauseated or vomiting? Do you have a feeling of fullness before you have really eaten very much? Or is the problem not having the energy to cook a nutritious meal? Sometimes people say they are just not hungry when they sit down to eat.

If the problem is related to nausea or vomiting, try using the suggestions in Chapter 4. If you are having a feeling of fullness, eating smaller meals more frequently instead of three big meals is helpful. It is definitely overwhelming to look at a full plate of food and think about eating everything. Another trick is to serve the food in an attractive way. Eat in the dining room with nice plates instead of in front of the television with paper plates. Playing your favorite music may make the meal feel like a more festive occasion. In this way, the meal will be more appealing, and you may be pleasantly surprised by how much you are able to eat.

In our society, mealtimes are often our times for socializing. Not being able to eat can have a negative meaning for many people. If you are unable to eat, it can feel unnatural. Make sure that you keep your mealtimes—and the times around them—as much as possible like they were before you were diagnosed with cancer. Returning to the usual ways of functioning may help to make the meal feel more normal. Being nervous or anxious can also upset your digestion. A return to some sense of normalcy may decrease your anxiety about food and eating.

When cancer and normal cells in our bodies die, they release substances into the body which can contribute to fatigue. Drinking enough fluid will help to flush out these waste byproducts and may make you feel less weary. Dehydration can also make you feel more fatigued, so drinking fluids will be beneficial either way.

When your fatigue is caused by an insufficient quantity or poor quality of sleep, look at your diet to make sure that you are not eating or drinking something which will keep you awake at night. Foods and drinks containing caffeine (chocolate, coffee, colas, and tea) should be avoided in the evening. If you are thirsty at bedtime, drinking an herbal tea or warm milk would be better.

Going to the bathroom frequently at night will also interrupt your sleep. If this is a problem, you might think about limiting how much you drink after dinner to avoid needing to urinate in the middle of the night. These simple suggestions may improve the quality and quantity of your rest at night.

Augmenting your diet with supplements may also be helpful. If your problem is due to a nutritional imbalance, you can take products, that are high in calories, protein, and other nutrients, such as Isocal and Ensure. If you have difficulty chewing or swallowing food, these supplements are easy to drink. If your fatigue is due to anemia, try to eat foods containing iron and vitamin C. Vitamin C helps you to absorb the iron you ingest. You might also check with your nurse or doctor about taking a multivitamin pill to enhance your diet.

Another dietary aid to help you sleep is a warm glass of milk before bed. You might remember your mother giving this to you when you were young. She was right! Foods such as warm milk or crackers and cheese have substances which help our brains to relax.

Finally, a dietary consultation with a registered dietician is often beneficial in providing guidance as to the best foods to eat if you are dealing with fatigue. The dietician can also help you to tailor your meals to your tastes. Your doctor or nurse can assist you in finding a dietician to speak with you.

Medications

Your doctor can prescribe medications for sleep if you need them, and a number of over-the-counter medicines are available as well. If you are thinking of taking a medication for sleep, ask your doctor or nurse. They can tell you whether there will be a problem with interactions between the other drugs you are already taking and the sleep medicines.

If your sleep is disturbed by pain or other symptoms, be sure to take the medicines prescribed for treatment of these problems. Once the pain or nausea is under control, you will be better able to rest.

Coping

Fatigue is a frequent complication of cancer and its treatments, and more than one factor may be contributing to the problem. Often, these factors are interrelated. The suggestions in this chapter for coping give you a range of alternatives, allowing you to experiment and discover what strategies work best for you.

10

Getting Support

by Jeff Kane, M.D.

Other people can be an important source of support when you are dealing with chemotherapy. You may need help with your basic physical requirements—a secure income, optimum home conditions, nutritious food, and adequate transportation. You may want to know where to find a decent wig or prosthesis. You may want to learn how to communicate more satisfactorily with those who treat you or hear how others handle the side effects of chemotherapy. You may want to learn about "alternative" nonmedical therapies. You may just want a shoulder to cry on, a sympathetic ear, or a hug. But whatever your support need is, it must come from other people.

Like many, you may be hesitant to ask for help. And many people do avoid seeking support. They have their reasons, and these are worth addressing.

"I feel that asking for help shows that I'm weak." Admittedly, asking for help means that you can't deal with the situation alone. But in how much of your life are you totally independent, anyway? When you think about it, almost all projects—raising a child, writing a book, building a home, or maintaining a business—are shared endeavors. Asking for help is a natural extension of the lifelong practice of applying assistance where and when it's needed. If you were to break your leg, you'd have a cast put on it; the cast doesn't announce that you're an incompetent person, simply that your body requires temporary support.

"Asking for help invites unwanted intimacy." You probably don't like to have your life invaded even by well-meaning people. People outside of your family don't really know how you like your food cooked or where your clothes get put away. If help means a part-time housekeeper or driver, you may see them as intruders. But once you understand that good help can be as therapeutic as medications, you'll begin to drop your resistance and eventually come to see this "intrusion" without resentment, if not as refreshingly welcome.

"I've always been the helper, asking for help just isn't who I am." This is a common sentiment among people dealing with illness. One hallmark of personal healing power, however, is the ability to see opportunity in every situation. The opportunity here, of course, is to broaden your behavioral repertoire— to become someone who helps *and* someone who can ask for help as well. Acknowledge your reluctance, take a deep breath, and ask anyway.

In any case, hesitancy in seeking help is ultimately based on your sense of how you relate to others. Now is as good a time as any to confront this sense and ask whether it remains helpful. People who do so often report improvement in the quality of their relationship.

Support People

Who is a "support person"? A support person is anyone who provides you help—who drives you to a treatment, brings you a glass of water, fills a prescription, or sits quietly with you. A support person may be a family member, friend, or caregiver, although sometimes those closest to you can be remarkably unsupportive. Instead of taking for granted that someone is or is not a support person, look instead to see if he or she exhibits qualities like these:

Love. The quality that's required here isn't the soppy, sentimental one that popular songs describe. What's needed is compassion, literally the ability to feel what another feels. Compassion generates a helping relationship, in which your support person emotionally comprehends your situation and sees it in the most positive and hopeful light.

For our purposes, regard love as attention: a support person's skill is equal to his or her use of attention. In this case, it's a measure of his or her ability to *listen*, or, more precisely, *sense* the messages you transmit.

Like other normal human beings, you are occasionally unconscious of deep feelings. A good listener will hear you, read your "body language," absorb your emotions like a sponge, and reflect them honestly back at you with a view toward your self-understanding.

Honesty. A good support person doesn't deal in wishful thinking or false cheer. Your most therapeutic friend will not necessarily be the one who offers you cures, rabidly slaps your back ("Honey, you look sooooo terrific!"), or feels sorry for you. Honesty usually requires little more than compassionate interest and a contentedness in just being with you.

A part of honesty is candidness. A supportive person encourages you and praises your strengths, to be sure, but also gently points out your weaknesses, those areas in which you could possibly make your life more comfortable. Those people who unfailingly flatter you will ultimately disappoint you, allowing you to persist in whatever nontherapeutic behavioral styles you have evolved over decades.

Centeredness. The perfect support person is one who can keep his or her perspective when you've lost yours. Consider how difficult it is for you to stay focused while your doctor gives you detailed and occasionally emotion-laden information. A good support person accompanies you, helps translate complexities, records information, asserts your preferences, and prompts you to remember the questions that you wanted to ask.

Humor. Don't leave home without it. Humor is one of humanity's most potent healing tools. If you lose yours, you'd better get a transfusion from your supporter's reservoir.

If you've compared your friends and relatives to this list of skills and are still confused about which of them might be your best support people, I suggest that you let your deeper mind guide you. Try this exercise.

1. Ensure that you'll have fifteen minutes of silence and privacy. Lie down and relax deeply.

2. Imagine yourself in an honest full-body view, looking as you do now. Notice detail and color in your mind's eye. Now begin to fill the space around this self-image with the images of people who seem to be carrying you, "supporting" you. You may or may not see your spouse, children, parents, or other relatives; you may see faces that surprise you. Now move back from this image, enlarging the visual field like a motion picture camera zooming back to a wider angle. See other figures a little farther from you—people who provide some support, but not as much as the primary figures.

3. What you've created is an image of your current support network as you understand it. Focus this image to

clarify details. Does a particular figure seem to be more supportive than you had thought? Does a figure seem absolutely unsupportive or even obstructive of the support of others?

4. Thank your imaginary supporters so that your next contacts with the actual people will be one in which your appreciation is obvious. Then let your images fade. Gradually, gently, open your eyes and sit up when ready.

5. Reviewing what you saw in this exercise, ask yourself which of those people you'd like to have more contact with. Are there others whom you might not want admitted to your hospital room?

Note that the qualities that define an ideal supporter are the same that define an ideal friend. Hopefully, you are a good friend to your supporters, as sensitive and honest with them as they are with you. Consider, then, that they can occasionally be tired or frazzled—poor prospects for immediate support. Human nature being what it is, they may say yes when for their own good they should say no. So try not to depend wholly on any one person, or even a few. Rotate your requests among a group you seek to enlarge.

In any case, strongly encourage your spouse or friends to take an occasional break. The physical and emotional burdens they bear are universally underestimated. So even if your spouse claims that he or she is ready to take on even more, work out a schedule with room for time off in it; even the most dedicated pal needs a night out once in awhile.

Support Groups

You can expect that your initial diagnosis will throw you and family members into emotional turmoil. If you find yourself anxious, depressed, angry, desperate, overwhelmed by other strong emotions, know that these are normal responses. The only way that they can affect you for the worse is if you repress them. So try to be honest in expressing your emotions, knowing that feelings like these regularly accompany cancer. If expressed, they will be *finite*: at any point in time, you have only so many tears.

Your family is your support group of first choice. Hopefully, you and family members can develop the tolerance, stamina, and flexibility to help each other ride out the emotional storms of the first few weeks. But if your family is not up to it in some way—or if you need an additional boost to your spirits—consider joining a cancer patient support group.

In the near future, support groups will be a standard component of cancer treatment, for they've been shown to be dramatically therapeutic. In one study at Stanford University, Dr. David Spiegel and his coworkers found that seriously ill cancer patients who participated in support groups stayed healthier significantly longer than their counterparts who hadn't joined groups. Indeed, the results were so striking that if a drug had achieved this result, the press would have hailed it as a "breakthrough."

That people can essentially be medicine to each other is exactly the point of support groups. Who know more about having—not diagnosing or treating, mind you, but having—cancer? Doctors or people with cancer?

Not long ago, when the word "cancer" was taboo, patients suffered alone, at home, unable to speak about it to others, even family members. Consequently, they experienced not only the symptoms of illness and treatment, but the frustration of social isolation as well. No one was there to tell them that emotional turbulence was a predictable side effect of the disease; many ended up scared or ashamed of their own feelings. They had no way of discussing important, naturally arising issues about life, sickness, and death with their peers. Very often they remained ignorant of even the simplest physical aids like wigs and prostheses.

By banding together in ever-increasing numbers of support groups throughout the country, cancer patients are pruning away these unnecessary miseries.

The common feature that members of cancer support groups share is the cancer experience. Members usually include people who have active cancer, some who are in remission, and some who have been in remission long enough to consider themselves cured. Most groups are facilitated by professionals or knowledgeable volunteers, but some are leaderless.

A support group is basically a small, caring community bonded by a deep fundamental experience. By their very nature, support groups tend to be accepting and gentle. Because members remember their own experience, they can anticipate shyness in those who are unaccustomed to speaking publicly of personal things.

Groups vary in general purpose. Some are professionally organized education sessions, covering topics like nutrition, chemotherapy, and self-care. Others serve primarily as information clearing houses, in which members share the latest in diagnostic and treatment methods. Many groups offer practice in coping skills, including meditation, visualization, stress management, and pain control. Some groups minimize their discussion of medical topics, leaning instead toward exploration and resolution of emotional issues.

In these latter groups, members speak of fears, triumphs, questions, and concerns. Not infrequently, they cry. More often, though, they laugh. As medical and emotional issues arise, participants discuss them from the perspective of their own personal histories. Advice giving is generally avoided, although a wealth of valuable information is likely to be discussed: what new medicine to ask the doctor about, which radiotherapy clinic offers more personable service, how to minimize side effects, deal with fatigue, decide on treatment options, learn of experimental treatment protocols, deal with the effect of one's cancer on coworkers, and so on.

A common side benefit of most groups is the deep friendship that can blossom between members because of the intimacy that an effective group shares.

People often underestimate the effect that their cancer has on those around them. Consequently, some groups welcome support people or are dedicated exclusively to them. If your supporters attend a group, expect them to have an experience parallel to yours. Resolution of their issues will create a more therapeutic relationship between them and you.

Before you seek a support group, determine what sort of group you want. Ask yourself these questions:

- Do you believe you would benefit from the company of other cancer patients?

- Are you looking for self-exploration, coping skills, contact with others, combinations of these, or information only?

- Do you have emotional needs unmet by your present support people?

- Would talking about your emotions help you, or do you think that it might be too intimate or threatening?

- Would you like your spouse or support person involved? If so, do you want her or him to join you in your group or in a separate one?

Two objections that commonly arise among people considering support groups require acknowledgment and response.

"I can't join a support group because public speaking makes me nervous." Speaking of personal matters within a group of relative strangers can obviously be threatening. But I've never come across a support group in which speaking is mandatory. These groups are, after all, dedicated not to tearing you down, but to building you up. It's always all right not to speak.

Indeed, much is to be gained simply by attending and listening to the stories of others. Soon you will find it difficult *not* to speak.

"I'm afraid that if I join a support group I'll be depressed by meeting people who are sicker than I am." This expectation is realistic: you probably *will* find people sicker than you. On the other hand, you will find people less sick than you. Consider that all your life you've seen people both sicker and less sick than you. This spectrum, a permanent part of the human condition, can and should remind you that you may get sicker, but you may come to feel better as well.

Finding a Support Group

First consult the obvious sources, like your doctor, a hospital social worker, and especially other patients. Most branches of the American Cancer Society try to maintain a current list of local support groups.

You will be put in touch with group organizers or facilitators. Ask them about aspects of their group relevant to your interests, such as discussion of feelings, information sharing, and coping-skills education. Don't forget to ask about mundane aspects such as fees, parking, and accessibility.

Groups vary not only in their overall goals, conduct, and membership, but also in style from meeting to meeting. If you're fortunate enough to live in an area with more than one group, try out several, and preferably go back more than once.

Founding a Support Group

If no support groups currently exist in your area, then it may be time to start one.

A cancer support group consists of, at the minimum, two cancer patients who want to talk with each other about their experience. If you don't know of such a person or can't find one through word-of-mouth, there are several routes to search.

Almost all cancer patients see medical doctors, so that's a place to start. Call your local oncologists' offices with your plan. Doctors are understandably reluctant to divulge the names and phone numbers of their patients, but they may be willing to post a notice of your intent.

Let the nearest branch of the American Cancer Society know you'd like to start a group. ACS offices routinely receive calls from people seeking existing groups, and have even been known to provide guidance and financial assistance.

If all else fails, consider going public. Try taking out a small classified ad in the "announcements" section of your local newspaper. Since you're offering a free service, many publications will run your ad free of charge. If you want to get fancier, send a brief announcement—including your name, phone number, and the title "Cancer Patient Support Group" in the return address—to a local radio station, asking that it be read as a public service announcement. Federal law requires radio stations to deliver a number of "PSAs" for nonprofit endeavors. If you do take a public route, keep in mind that you'll be dealing with the public-at-large. Expect to receive some responses unrelated to cancer support.

Operating a Support Group

Design your group carefully. Here are several issues to consider.

Numbers. How many people will you limit your group to? More than eight or ten regular members will make for an unwieldy group that minimizes individual input. If a large number of members keep returning, consider splitting into manageable units.

Time. How often will you meet and for how long? Balance your enthusiasm with people's limited energy. Most support groups meet either weekly or biweekly for ninety minutes to two hours.

Location. Find a mutually convenient place that's accessible to people who are debilitated or in wheelchairs. Consider ease of parking, night-lighting, rest room facilities, distance to the meeting room, adequate number of comfortable chairs, and so on. To save yourselves headaches, avoid having the group meet in members' homes, at least at first. Churches, libraries, and certain businesses are often happy to let support groups use rooms free during off-hours, and a neutral setting will give you a chance to determine the makeup of the group and its needs.

Membership. Is the group open only to people with active cancer? Is it open to people in remission? People who consider themselves cured, but still have feelings to deal with? People who have an out-of-town relative with cancer? People who haven't had cancer, but are frightened of it? People who simply want to learn more about it?

Will the group be for women only? Men only? You may wish to limit your group to people with a particular kind of cancer (for example, women's breast cancer support groups are becoming more numerous).

Do you know of anyone interested in beginning a support group for those who are not appropriate for your group?

I suggest that you keep the membership of the group as unrestrictive as possible. You are likely to find that the group's membership and its interests will benefit from a degree of flexibility.

Emphasis. Cancer support groups flourish with many different areas of focus. One prominent self-help center emphasizes art therapy techniques for self-understanding within the experience of cancer. Another program teaches techniques for attaining inner peace. Another group features a different speaker each week; members have heard psychotherapists, nutritionists, dream workers, meditation teachers, and a host of other specialists. Still another takes each meeting as it comes, dealing with extremely varied issues at each meeting.

Do you want only discussion among members, or do you want other features—like teaching of pain control and meditation—as well? Do you want your group leaderless or led by a skilled facilitator? Are you willing to incur shared expenses?

The flavor you'll want in your meetings depends entirely on the interests of members. Most members will never have been in support groups before, so there's ample opportunity for you to experiment.

For orientation, consider looking at the way established programs conduct their groups. Here are a few sources of information.

American Cancer Society
1599 Clifton Road N.E.
Atlanta, GA 30322
(Ask for their publication "Guidelines on Self-Help and Mutual Support Groups.")

Center for Attitudinal Healing
19 Main Street
Tiburon, CA 94920

"Common Concern" Program of California Department of Mental Health
Coordinator's Manual Published by New Harbinger Publications
5674 Shattuck Avenue
Oakland, CA 94609

Creighton Health Institute
275 Elliot Drive
Menlo Park, CA 94025

Exceptional Cancer Patient ("ECaP") Program
1302 Chapel Street
New Haven, CT 06511

The Wellness Community
1235 5th Street

Santa Monica, CA 90401

Y-ME
1-800-221-2141
National breast cancer support hotline. Has chapters in
Chicago; Palm Beach, FL; Washington, DC; Santa Barbara, CA; and in Arkansas.

However you formulate your group, do try to stay informal. If you don't, you may end up tape-recording sessions, keeping records, electing officers, and perhaps even operating by par-
liamentary procedure. This kind of structure is grotesquely far
from the original intent, which is for people in similar situations
simply to be with each other.

Beyond Support Groups

Once you start reaping the therapeutic fruits of support, whether
from individuals or groups, you may want to ask yourself a far-
reaching question: How can I make *all* my relationships supportive? Indeed, why should you not live in a permanent atmo-
sphere of support? Once you seriously consider this possibility,
you will instinctively steer your life toward it.

Everyone whose life has been touched by cancer share one
common perception: the revelation that time is limited. Some
people are overflowing with support; others operate otherwise.
It becomes natural, then, to ask, "How can I maximize the time
I spend with the people who support me?"

In the end, the answer is obvious. And without even thinking consciously about it, you'll find yourself moving toward supportive people and away from unsupportive ones.

In one way this process is painful, for no one likes to leave
old friends. But at the same time, every departure entails a des-
tination. Your adventures in seeking support will lead you
toward a self-image in which your development, your understanding, and your peace become a joyful priority.

About the Author

Jeff Kane, M.D., devotes his practice to counseling people with chronic and life-threatening illnesses. He has expressed his views on illness as a consultant, workshop leader, community college instructor, radio talk show host, and hatha-yoga teacher. He is the author of *Be Sick Well: A Healthy Approach to Chronic Illness* (New Harbinger Publications, Inc., 1991) as well as many published articles. He also facilitates the Cancer Support Group at Sutter Memorial Hospital in Sacramento, California.

11

Relaxation and Stress Reduction

Your body tenses and makes adrenaline when you're faced with a threat. This stress response is designed to help you survive danger; it's a warning for you to flee or fight. But when stress becomes chronic, it dampens your immune system and makes it harder for your body to heal.

It's important while on chemotherapy to do everything in your power to keep your immune system strong. Relaxation techniques can not only help you feel less overwhelmed, but also help you reduce the immunity-suppressing effects of stress. Breathing, muscle relaxation, and imagery techniques, as well as self-hypnosis, can assist you to relax your body. Other techniques such as thought stopping and systematic desensitization can help you deal with specific fears.

Deep Breathing

Deep breathing is an ancient Eastern technique as well as a modern, medically proven adjunct to Western medicine. It oxygenates your blood while releasing muscle tension in your diaphragm. Deep breathing is an excellent way to achieve very rapid relaxation. It will help you feel better in a hurry when you're facing some immediate stress.

If you want to practice deep breathing, try lying down in a comfortable place. Bend your knees and lay one hand on your abdomen and the other on your chest. Breathe lightly through your nose. In this normal breathing pattern, the hand on your chest and the hand on your abdomen will rise and fall together. But in deep breathing, only the hand on your abdomen will rise, while your chest will move very slightly, if at all. By pushing your breath way down into your abdomen, you not only get more air, but you also stretch your diaphragm so that the tense abdominal muscles can start to relax.

Now try it. Breathe deeply so that only the hand on your abdomen rises with the breath. Breathe in slowly through your nose, pushing up the hand, and then exhale through your mouth. Sometimes it feels good to make a whooshing noise as you let go of the breath.

When you feel ready, take another breath. Breathe only when you feel like it. You're taking in a lot more air, so you'll breathe more slowly than usual. If you rush it and breathe faster than you need to, you're going to get too much oxygen, and you may feel a little dizzy. If that happens, just concentrate on slowing your breathing so that you take a breath *only when you need to.*

If you have trouble pushing up the hand on your abdomen and only the hand on your chest seems to move, then you need more practice. One thing you can do is push down with the hand on your abdomen. While you're pushing down on your abdomen, try to use a deep breath to push it back up.

Practice the deep breathing technique until you feel comfortable with it; until it feels easy, almost second nature. You should set aside three or four times during the day to work on your breathing. When you've mastered deep breathing while lying down, practice it sitting in a chair, feet flat on the floor, hands resting on your knees. You'll find the practice comes in handy because deep breathing is an extremely effective way of dealing with the tension you may feel while having an IV started or having your blood drawn in the lab.

Autogenic Breathing

Deep breathing can be combined with imagery for extremely effective stress relief. To learn autogenic breathing, start by lying down and doing deep breathing for two to three minutes. When you're in a comfortable rhythm and feeling more relaxed, visualize yourself lying on a warm, white beach. Feel the warmth from the sun caress your skin, radiate into your muscles, and finally your bones. Feel the soft, warm breeze touch your body.

Now imagine being covered with warm sand; the weight of the sand feels like a warm, protective hand on your body. Feel the heavy warmth penetrate deep into your muscles, relaxing and purifying your body. The warmth and the heaviness relax your body more and more deeply.

Now listen to the ebb and flow of your breath. Say to yourself, "warm" as your breath comes in and then "heavy" as your breath goes out. Warm on the in-breath, heavy on the out-breath. Warm and heavy, warm and heavy. Really try to feel the warmth in your limbs as you say "warm" on the in-breath. Try to visualize the heavy sand holding your body safe and secure as you breathe out.

Stay on the beach as long as your want, letting the autogenic breathing relax and refresh your body. Practice the imagery until the warmth and heaviness are easy to feel. Practicing this technique at home can pay off later when you're having your chemotherapy. The imagery can help you to relax even during extended IV treatments.

Other Relaxation Imagery

Visualization is a lovely way to take a break, a vacation from stress. You can go anywhere in your mind, creating a retreat of exquisite peace and beauty. The following three "retreats" will give you an idea of the special places you can go without ever leaving your chair. With just a little practice, you can start designing your own retreat that has all the elements you need for deep relaxation.

Retreat 1

It's dark and cool as you begin the path leading upward toward the mountain. Early morning stars and the moon guide you along this trail beside a rushing stream. Slowly you climb, step by step, along the flowered path wet with morning dew. The sky lightens into a pale blue. You know this day will be warm. Cardinals, bluebirds, and wrens start to whistle and sing, keeping you company along the path that begins to open into stands of pine and oak. You walk on, feeling strong and happy that you are alive and eager to stand atop the mountain at sunrise. The stream next to the path trickles over a tiny falls. You place your hand under it, drinking its clear, cold water. You go on. Your body feels light and strong as you climb. The first red rays of sunlight are just peeking out to your left as the trail reaches the edge of a granite knoll. You're at the top now, and the sun breaks behind the mountain range on the horizon, rising quickly, an enormous ball of power greeting you, warming you, lighting you. You sit on a rock, breathe deeply, inhale the clean, crisp air. In the valley below, you can see rivers of mist flowing. But here the warm, bright sun shines above you, strengthening you as it does the plants and the birds. Here at the top, you feel a sense of peace and relaxation flowing throughout your entire body.

Retreat 2

You awake slowly in your room by the ocean. Darkness envelopes you as you put on your beach slippers and pad out to the screen porch, warm cup in hand. You sit in the rocker, quietly rocking back and forth, listening to the roar of the cresting sea. The stars pierce the sky's black blanket. You breathe quietly, deeply, feeling the rolling of the rocker on the wooden floor. Near the shore, long grasses wave gently, mocking the movement of the sea. You are safe. The moist air caresses your face. The warm drink soothes. The sky lightens, and the stars disappear. You see for miles. The sun rises red over the sea line as pelicans glide between the troughs of the soft sea swells. Light glows, bathing you. You continue to breathe deeply, slowly, mirroring the rhythm of the waves as they run up the shore.

Retreat 3

The weeks have been hectic, but you are safe now on the train. You sink deeply into your seat and watch the vast, pale desert slip past the train window. Buttes stand silent and orange above the sagebrush-covered ground. The sun is setting, and the sky flames red and purple. The light fades slowly, but you can still see the mountains cut against the night sky. The low, rocking thunder of the train wheels blankets all other sounds. You feel safe, peaceful as the train rocks gently under you. You sink more deeply into your seat as you hear the clacking wheels. You have no problems to solve, nothing to think about as the train carries you through the desert night. It holds you, rocking gently as it speeds.

Your retreat may be nothing like these. You may call up a room from childhood, the breakfast table at your grandmother's house, a Paris cafe, a sandbar at the bend of a river, a high meadow, a campground beneath whispering trees. Go there often; use your retreat when you feel anxious and tired, when you are uncomfortable, when you are bored.

Imagery and Healing

Imagery is a powerful tool that can do far more than relax you. Imagery can also help you to heal. O. Carl Symonton, in his book, *Getting Well Again* (J. P. Tarcher, Inc., 1978), shows how certain kinds of imagery may increase your ability to fight cancer. Symonton encourages people to imagine ferocious white blood cells tearing and consuming the weak cancer cells. Or you can visualize the chemotherapy as a powerful chemical that surrounds and destroys cancer cells. Symonton believes that *how* you visualize the cancer, the chemotherapy, and the white cells is very important. Read his book to learn more about how his use of visualization can help you.

While Symonton's techniques are widely used, there are many other approaches to healing visualizations. Many people use images of white light that soothes and heals a specific body area. Samples of healing visualizations can be found in *Visualization for Change* by Patrick Fanning (New Harbinger Publications, 1988). A sample script and instructions for making your own visualization tape are included in Chapter 12.

Progressive Muscle Relaxation

Progressive muscle relaxation (PMR) is a technique developed in the 1920s by Dr. Edmund Jacobson. It is based on the theory that a person cannot be both relaxed and anxious at the same time. To calm anxiety, muscles are progressively tightened and released in sequence throughout your entire body.

In the beginning, PMR takes fifteen to twenty minutes for each practice session. But in a few weeks, after you learn it thoroughly, you can tighten groups of muscles simultaneously and reduce the time spent to a few minutes. When using this technique, avoid tensing muscles or areas of your body that may be painful. If pain is a problem, just read this section to learn PMR sequences, and then go on to the next section, "Relaxation Without Tension," to use this technique in a safer way.

Basic PMR Procedure

First tighten your right fist and forearm. Clench as hard as you can for seven seconds. Notice what the tension feels like. Now release your fist and feel the muscles in your forearm relax for twenty seconds. Notice how relaxation feels—heavy or warm or tingly. Really experience the relaxation in your hand and forearm. Repeat the procedure with your right fist once again, always noticing as you relax the release of the tension. Now do the same thing with your left fist and forearm. Tense for seven seconds and relax for twenty. Now do both fists at the same time, tensing for seven seconds and relaxing for twenty. Always notice how relaxation feels in your muscles.

The next step is to tense the muscles in your right arm. Make them as hard as you can for seven seconds and then relax. Do the tensing and relaxing twice with each arm.

As you continue through the exercise, tighten each specific muscle for seven seconds and relax for twenty. And then repeat the same muscle once again. Pay attention to what relaxation feels like in each muscle.

Now focus on your face, the seat of so much tension. Wrinkle up your forehead. Hold it taut, then release.

Now frown and squint your eyes, holding them tightly shut. Release.

Purse your mouth into an O. Relax and notice what it's like to let go of tension in this area of your face.

Now tighten your jaw, bite hard, and push your tongue against the roof of your mouth. Relax and notice what it feels like to release the tension in your jaw.

Turning to the neck and shoulder area, press your head back against your chair and then relax your head. Roll slowly and gently to the right and then to the left.

Straighten your head and gently let it fall forward. Relax and really feel the release of tension in your neck.

Now hunch your shoulders. Relax and let them droop, feeling the relaxation spread through your neck, throat, and shoulders.

Feel the relaxation move throughout your entire body. Feel the comfort of the heaviness. Now breathe in and fill your lungs completely. Hold your breath and notice the tension. As you exhale, feel all tension leaving your body. Repeat the full breath several times, paying attention to how tension can drain out of your body as you exhale.

Tighten your abdominal muscles, just as if you were preparing to be punched. When you relax, let the tension drain away again. Put your hand on your belly and push it up with a deep breath. As you let go, feel your entire abdomen relax.

Gently arch your back slightly. Be careful not to strain it. Relax again and take another deep breath.

Tighten the muscles in your lower back. Relax and notice how the muscles feel without tension.

Tighten your buttocks and thighs. Flex your thighs by pressing down your heels as hard as you can. Relax and notice what it's like to let go of tension in these big muscles.

Now curl your toes downward, making your calves tense. Relax.

Now pull your toes back toward your face, creating tension in your shins. Relax again. Observe the muscles in your feet and calves. Notice how it feels for them finally to relax.

Just feel the heaviness throughout your lower body as relaxation deepens. Notice the relaxation in your feet, ankles, calves, shins, knees, thighs, and buttocks. Let the relaxation spread to your stomach, lower back, and chest. Let it become deeper and deeper. Experience the relaxation deepening in your shoulders, neck, arms, and hands. Then experience the feeling of looseness and relaxation in your neck, jaw, and all your facial muscles. Your whole body feels more and more deeply relaxed.

Shorthand PMR Procedure

After you've practiced PMR for several weeks and are aware of the effects of tension and relaxation on specific muscles, you're ready to shorten the process. You can now tighten and relax certain muscle groups simultaneously. Just as you did before, tighten for seven seconds and relax for twenty, but be sure to avoid painful areas or straining. Carefully observe the effects of both the contraction and the relaxation of your muscles. As your muscles loosen, let your whole body grow heavy and still.

1. Curl your fists. Tighten your biceps and forearms (in a Charles Atlas pose). Relax.

2. Wrinkle your forehead. At the same time, press your head as far back as possible, rolling it clockwise in a complete circle. Reverse the direction of the roll. Now wrinkle up the muscles of your face like a walnut. Frown with your eyes squinted, lips pursed, tongue pressed against the roof of your mouth. And with the same walnut face, hunch your shoulders. Relax.

3. Breathe deeply into your abdomen as you slightly arch your back. Hold, observe, and relax. Breathe deeply again, pressing out your abdomen. Hold. And then relax.

4. Now curl your toes while simultaneously tightening your calf, thigh, and buttocks muscles. Relax. Pull your feet and toes back toward your face, tightening your shins. Hold and relax.

Relaxation Without Tension

This exercise involves relaxing your muscles in the same sequence that you learned with PMR. But there's one difference:

you don't tighten each muscle. Instead, you notice any tension that may exist in the muscle and then "relax away" the tightness.

Twice a day practice going though each muscle in the PMR sequence and "relaxing away" any tension you find. Try to make the muscle feel as relaxed as it did right after you let go in the PMR exercise.

Relaxation without tension allows you to scan your body for hot spots of tightness. There's no embarrassing process that others might observe. You can relax away tension in the doctor's office or the clinic. You can use this technique to relax away tension while you're receiving chemotherapy.

Self-Hypnosis

This is an extremely effective technique for relaxing your body and strengthening your mind. You can use hypnosis to seed affirmations and positive thoughts that will help you get through having an IV started, chemotherapy, and other treatment procedures. Self-hypnosis makes you relax in the moment. Through the power of suggestion, it also helps you relax long after the trance state has ended. When you suggest to yourself during hypnosis that you'll feel more calm or confident during a particularly stressful procedure, the chances are that you really will feel that way. Here's how you do it.

To induce hypnosis, plan for a twenty-minute session. Loosen your clothing and lie or sit in a comfortable place. Select words such as "relax" or "peaceful and strong" that you can repeat mentally during the induction. These will be cue words that help you to deepen your level of relaxation. Before starting the induction, you should also choose an affirmation or suggestion for your subconscious to carry into the future, when you're facing stressful procedures (see the list of affirmations later in this chapter for suggestions).

Close your eyes and feel them begin to get heavy. Take a deep breath, way down into your abdomen. And as you exhale, feel the relaxation spread throughout your entire body. Take another deep breath, and as you exhale say to yourself your cue word or phrase that will deepen the relaxation.

Now begin to focus on your legs. Imagine that they have become heavy lead weights. Tell yourself that your legs are becoming heavier and heavier, more and more deeply relaxed. Just repeat the phrases: "Heavier and heavier, heavy and letting go, heavy and relaxed, more and more deeply relaxed."

When you achieve a sense of heaviness in your legs, turn your attention to your arms. Your arms, too, can become heavier and heavier, heavy and relaxed, becoming more and more deeply relaxed as you feel them letting go. Just repeat these phrases in any combination until your arms truly begin to feel heavy. Then repeat the same phrases for both your arms and your legs.

Now turn your attention to your face. Suggest to yourself that your forehead is becoming as smooth as silk, smooth and relaxed. Your cheeks, too, are smooth and relaxed. Your forehead and cheeks are more and more deeply relaxed, letting go of tension, feeling smooth and relaxed. Repeat these phrases until you feel that your face has let go of all muscular tension.

Now focus on your jaw. Suggest that your jaw is becoming loose and relaxed. Suggest that as your jaw becomes more and more deeply relaxed, you'll feel the muscles letting go and your lips beginning to part. Repeat the phrase "loose and relaxed" until you feel your jaw let go of tension.

Now turn your attention to your neck and shoulders. Suggest that your neck is centered and relaxed. Your shoulders are relaxed and drooping. Take a slow breath and let the relaxation deepen in your neck and shoulders.

Take another deep breath, and as you exhale let the relaxation spread into your chest and stomach and back. Take several more deep breaths. As you exhale, let the feelings of relaxation deepen in your torso.

Now it's time to go to a special place. A place of safety and peace. It may be at the beach or on a mountaintop or maybe a room from your childhood. It may be a place where you always felt loved and accepted. Your special place can be a real location or something entirely made up. In a moment you'll walk there. You can imagine reaching your special place by descending a flight of stairs or walking down a forest path or entering a gate. In ten steps you'll be there. With each step you'll grow more and more deeply relaxed, feeling peaceful and safe as you move toward your special place.

Now you will grow more relaxed with each step: ten ... nine ... eight ... seven ... six ... five ... four ... three ... two ... one ... zero. (If you want to go through the countdown two or even three times to deepen hypnosis, that's perfectly fine.)

Now in your special place you can further deepen the feelings of relaxation. The following suggestions can be made in any order. Repeat them over and over again, until you reach a state of deep calm.

- Drifting deeper and deeper, deeper and deeper.
- More and more drowsy, peaceful, and calm.
- Drifting and drowsy, drowsy and drifting.
- Drifting down, down, down into total relaxation.

After you've given yourself these deepening suggestions, let yourself relax and enjoy your special place. Now is a good time to repeat the suggestion or affirmation that you've prepared before hypnosis. Suggestions that others have used include affirmations like these.

- I am feeling stronger each day.
- I can relax during the chemotherapy.
- The chemotherapy will make me healthier and healthier.
- The cancer is dying; the chemotherapy is killing it.
- I feel strengthened by the love of my friends and family.
- I can relax and let the chemotherapy work.

Once you've repeated your suggestion or affirmation several times, you can bring yourself up to normal consciousness any time you wish. To come all the way up, simply count from one to ten. After you get to around five, suggest to yourself that you're getting more and more alert, refreshed, and wide awake. Keep making these suggestions as you count the remaining numbers and begin opening your eyes around the count of nine.

Don't try to drive or do anything that requires focused attention immediately after hypnosis. Relax for a little while longer and enjoy the feelings of calm that hypnosis usually brings.

Thought Stopping

When someone says, "Chemotherapy makes me nervous," this statement makes sense intuitively. But it isn't really true. It isn't chemotherapy that makes people nervous. Rather, the anxiety results from a series of *thoughts* and *worries* about chemotherapy. If you can pay attention to what you say to yourself about the things that scare you, you will see how your thoughts can add to your anxiety. Here is a list of some of the things that one man thought just before treatment.

- How many times will they have to stick me today before they get the IV right?
- I wonder how sick I'll feel?
- I hate the whole procedure, I hate sitting here.
- What if I feel really weak?
- I wonder if I'm going to be able to keep working.
- These drugs are too strong; maybe they'll do more harm than good.

These thoughts, and a host of others like them, had made him nervous. Each frightening thought triggered the production of adrenaline, which only increased his feelings of anxiety and set off another round of scary thoughts. This process is known as the *anxiety feedback loop*: thoughts anticipating danger or pain cause the body to produce adrenaline. The adrenaline, in turn, stimulates the lymbic area of your brain so that you feel anxious. The anxiety seems to confirm your sense of danger, which then stimulates more thoughts of pain and catastrophe. The feedback loop can keep your anxiety spiraling upward till you feel tremendously upset.

Breaking the Loop

Thought stopping is an important technique for interrupting the feedback loop. If you shut off the frightening thoughts and the adrenaline surge that each thought triggers, you can start to calm down.

Here's how it works. Whenever you feel anxious, check to see what you're thinking. Notice if you're anticipating pain or problems—anything that's scary. Then shout "Stop!" to yourself. Just really scream it internally. You need to make the "Stop!" loud so that you can interrupt the flow of fear-provoking thoughts. If you can't interrupt the thoughts by commanding them to stop, you'll need something more imperative. Clap your hands or shout out loud (if no one's around to hear you). Or snap a rubber band around your wrist—the sharp sting will help to break the chain of thoughts.

Stop and Breathe

Once you've stopped the thoughts, you'll need something to replace them. Nature hates a vacuum; the negative thoughts will soon return if nothing fills the gap. You've already learned deep breathing. As soon as you interrupt the flow of thoughts, start taking slow, deep breaths. Really try to stretch and relax your diaphragm. Focus all your attention on your breathing, feeling its warmth permeate your body.

Now count your breaths. On each exhalation count, "One … two … three … four." After your fourth exhalation, start over again with one. Focus on the counting until your inner talk falls still, your anxiety lessens, and your mind becomes peaceful.

After you finish counting your breaths, don't worry if negative thoughts come back again. They frequently do. Immediately counter them by shouting "Stop!" and beginning to focus on your breathing. Count your breaths for one or two minutes and see if you're feeling calmer. Some people have to stop anxious thoughts over and over again as they anticipate their next chemotherapy treatment. That's okay. The important thing is not to let the anxious thoughts take root, not to dwell on them. Each anxious thought you stop protects you from a burst of adrenaline and a subsequent increase in your nervousness. This is hard work, but it pays off big dividends by lowering your overall stress level.

Affirmations

In addition to counting your breaths, you can replace frightening thoughts with positive affirmations. An affirmation is a short, pithy statement that helps you feel more self-confident and stronger and less fearful.

Here is a list of affirmations that you may use. Choose a few that you like and memorize them. Or use them for ideas to create unique affirmations of your own.

About relaxation

- Relaxation floods my body like a healing golden light.

- Each breath brings a flood of healing power to every corner of my body.

- I am filled with peace, calm, and serenity.

- Relaxation, enjoyment, and love are the things that keep me well.

- Taking care of myself keeps me strong.

- Relaxation is the gift I give myself.
- Every time I breathe in, I bring a wave of peace and relaxation. Every time I breathe out, I let go of tension and fear.

To reduce fear about treatments

- I can get through this.
- I can take care of myself.
- I can ask for what I need.
- The people around me (my nurse, my doctor, my family) know how to make sure that I am safe and comfortable.
- Every chemotherapy treatment takes me another step towards health and recovery.
- Cancer cells are weak and sick and confused.
- Chemotherapy is a strong ally. It works with my body's natural defenses to wipe out the defective cancer cells.
- I am open to the healing power of the medications.

After chemotherapy treatment

- The chemotherapy has done its job. Now it will be washed out of my body, taking with it the dead cancer cells.
- My body's natural defenses are building again and will be ready to protect me again.
- Chemotherapy is like a great crashing wave. It may shake me up for a minute, but now the water has receded, and I am safe again on the shore.
- Chemotherapy is like a torrential downpour, washing away the weak and broken cancer cells, leaving the strong healthy cells glistening in the sun.

- Chemotherapy has been like allied troops coming to a troubled area, routing the enemy, then returning the region to peace and beauty and health.

Systematic Desensitization

Some people are tremendously afraid of needles; some fear the symptoms or sensations surrounding chemotherapy. If you have strong fears about IVs or the chemotherapy experience, deep breathing and muscle relaxation may not be enough to achieve calm. Fortunately, there is a highly effective method for dealing with strong fears that you can use on your own or with the help of a counselor. *Systematic desensitization* was developed in the 1950s by Joseph Wolpe and has had an excellent 40-year track record of helping people overcome fear.

Systematic desensitization allows you to imagine scenes of higher and higher levels of anxiety while maintaining complete physical relaxation. You move incrementally, scene by scene, from the least anxiety-evoking to the most stressful situation you can imagine. One emotion (relaxed calm) is used to counteract another (anxiety). Even the most threatening situations can be gotten used to—if you do it gradually, step by step.

Here's what you do. Everything in systematic desensitization depends on constructing an appropriate *hierarchy*. This is a list of stressful situations that ranges from almost no anxiety to the highest level of fear. To construct your hierarchy, imagine having to deal with the chemotherapy experience. Think first about the least threatening part of it, perhaps imagining your self removed in space or time from the whole situation. Low-stress items on your hierarchy might include dressing to go to the clinic or even making an appointment for your chemotherapy treatments. Items that are more anxiety evoking would place you closer in time or space to the experience. For you, these experiences might include checking in with the receptionist at the clinic or having the nurse wipe your arm with alcohol before inserting the IV. Items at the top end of the hierarchy would be the part of the experience you fear most. This might be the needle stick or the sensation of the drug entering your veins or a particular side effect.

Go ahead now and try to develop your own scenes for a hierarchy. You need between eight and twenty scenes. Some people like to write the scenes down randomly, just as they come to mind. Others put the least scary scene at the top of a piece of paper and the most frightening one at the bottom. Then they try to fill in six or more scenes of graduated intensity in between. However you do it, when you've finally thought of enough scenes for an eight- to twenty-item hierarchy, put them in order down a page from the least to most stressful.

Here's a sample hierarchy from a 43-year-old woman who was facing her first chemotherapy treatment.

1. Thinking about going for treatment.

2. Preparing for treatment—shopping and preparing meals in advance, arranging childcare, arranging my work schedule.

3. Going to the lab for blood tests two days before chemotherapy.

4. Waking up on the morning of the day of the treatment.

5. Riding to the clinic.

6. Checking in with the receptionist.

7. Sitting in the waiting room.

8. Undressing in the exam room and waiting for the doctor.

9. Waiting in the treatment area for my turn.

10. Watching the nurse prepare the IV bags, tubing, and syringes.

11. Preparing to have the IV started—the feel of the tourniquet, the smell of alcohol.

12. Having the needle inserted and feeling the medicine going into my veins.

Notice that each item on the hierarchy is a little more stressful than the one before it. The important thing is to make the hierarchy *graduated* so that there is only a small increase in anxiety level from item to item.

Desensitization Procedure

Once you've developed your hierarchy, it's time to start using it. Here's what you do.

Relax. Start each desensitization session by taking ten to fifteen minutes to relax. Use deep breathing and progressive muscle relaxation to make your body as free of stress as possible.

Visualize a peaceful scene. Use the special place that you imagined while practicing hypnosis or think of a place where you feel safe, calm, and peaceful. It could be in the mountains or the beach, real or imagined, indoors or outdoors. It doesn't matter as long as you can vividly create the image. Practice visualizing the scene right now. See the shapes and colors, hear the sounds, feel the texture, the temperature. Make the scene and feelings as real and detailed as possible.

Start the first scene of your hierarchy. After you feel really relaxed, switch from your peaceful place to the first scene of your hierarchy. This scene, too, should be as vivid as possible. Create as much detail as you can so that it feels as if you're right there. Don't picture yourself feeling any particular emotion; just imagine the situation. Should you feel any anxiety, stop the image immediately and return to your peaceful place. If you don't feel anxiety, continue to visualize this first item from your hierarchy for thirty seconds. When you can visualize a scene twice without anxiety, go on to the next item on your hierarchy.

What to do between scenes. When you've stopped visualizing a scene from your hierarchy—either because you feel anxious or you've visualized it for the full thirty seconds—take a deep breath and return to your peaceful scene. Do the relaxation-without-tension exercise described earlier in this chapter. Focus on each of your muscle groups in sequence, relaxing away any tension that you find. When you feel calm and relaxed, go back to your hierarchy.

Progress through your hierarchy. Never stay in a scene that makes you anxious. Cut it off immediately and return to the peaceful place. If one scene continues to make you anxious time after time, skip it and work it in farther up your hierarchy. It's probably more anxiety-provoking than you thought and belongs up with the more stressful items. Make your first desensitization session no more than fifteen or twenty minutes. Later sessions can be stretched to as much as half an hour. Expect to master no more than two or three scenes in each session. If you find that your anxiety is high for every scene, it probably means that you need to relax more deeply—both at the onset and during the interval between hierarchy scenes. If you put more time into the relaxation process, you may find that you desensitize more quickly to the frightening images.

When you finish. When you complete your hierarchy, expect your anxiety to be improved but not absent. Chemotherapy IVs may no longer be overwhelming, but they won't be a walk in the park either. The important thing is that you *can* reduce your anxiety. You can reduce it to a point where you're able to cope and get through the experience.

12

Scripts for Relaxation and Visualization Tapes
Body Relaxed—Mind at Ease

by Harriett Sanders, L.C.S.W.

How To Use the Scripts

To obtain maximum benefit from the two scripts, it is best to either have them recorded or read aloud by another to you. In either case the scripts should be narrated in a slow, soothing relaxing tone, with ample time allowed for the formation of images and follow through with other suggestions. When making your own tape, you may wish to use pleasant background music. Just make sure that any music you record does not overpower or compete with the narration.

The relaxation and visualization scripts given here are designed to be used together—with the relaxation script providing the lead-in to the visualization script. They may, however, be used separately. When using the relaxation script alone, be sure to allow time at the end to come out of the relaxed state. You may want to include a modification of the last paragraph of the visualization script or other similar suggestions that would gradually lead you back into an awakened state.

Use the scripts as frequently as you like. The more you use them, the easier the process will become for you and undoubtedly the more beneficial the results will be. Using the script in the middle of the day can provide a refreshing break and at bedtime a delightful prelude to a restful night's sleep. Listening to the script before, during, or after treatment is highly recommended to offset stress, anxiety, or discomfort.

You may either sit in a chair or lie down when listening to the tape or having the script read to you. The ideal position is simply the one that works best for you. Feel free to experiment. Find a comfortable place to relax—one that is quiet and where you will not be disturbed. Dim the lights. Settle in and ENJOY!

Relaxation Script

And now it is time to become still and relax. Time to turn within, to journey to that special place deep inside you that knows only peace; only comfort; only calm. Find a comfortable position in your chair. You may want to rest your hands gently in your lap or on your knees or let your arms just dangle at your sides. There is no right or wrong way to relax, just whatever feels right for you. If you haven't already done so you may want to gently close your eyes, letting the closing of your eyes be a signal to the outside world that, for this next little while, you are going to detach, to let go, to turn within. Let go of all tension and strain. This is not a time to be thinking about outer concerns, stresses, or worries. This is a time just to be still. Still your body now and quiet your thoughts. Throughout this entire exercise, know that you will always be in control, that there is nothing to fear. So let go now. Allow your mind and body to be at rest and gently release into the calm.

Focus now on your breathing. For the next few breaths, breathe in slowly and deeply, through your nose and, at the top of the inhale, hold it—and now breathe out softly and slowly through your mouth. Once again, breathe in, slowly, through your nose, hold it—now breathe out, gradually and softly, through your mouth. As you exhale now, experience the flow of your breath as it gently and evenly exits your body; feel that wonderful sense of stillness and peace that comes as you release. Once more now, breathe in, slowly, through your nose, hold it— now breathe out, gradually and slowly, through your mouth. Breathe normally now, without effort, without strain—just let your body follow the natural rhythm, the natural cadence set by your breathing and allow it to move you deeper and deeper into the calm. Should you find any outer thoughts attempting to intrude and compete with this state of peace that is engulfing you now, just let these thoughts gently pass through and then fade away into nothingness. Let them go. If you find yourself beginning to nod off to sleep, or if the sound of my voice trails in and trails out, that's okay. Whatever works for you will be just fine. So just relax and let go. Any outer noise, any outer distraction that you might hear will only serve to move you far- ther and farther away and deeper and deeper into the calm. Now focus again on your breathing, and this time, as you inhale, I want you to silently say to yourself the word *let*, and as you exhale silently, say the word *go*. Breathing in: *let*, breathing out: *go. Let go. Let go. Let go.* It is okay to let go. It is safe to let go. For it is in letting go of all outer stresses, all tension, all distress and *dis-ease*, it is in the letting go of these experiences that you open to the healing your body so desperately needs for the restoration to health and wholeness. So fear not, resist not, just let go. All is well.

Now feel this relaxing sense of calm beginning to invade your body. I want you to imagine this beautiful sense of relaxation, imagine it being a white, puffy cloud of light that begins to ascend your body at your feet. Feel this beautiful cloud of light as it moves in and between your toes, allow it to travel along the soles of your feet, up into your heels and into your ankles. Just feel both your feet now immersed in this soft, billowy cloud of light. Feel all the tightness in your feet beginning now to dissipate, as your muscles relax and let go—leaving you with the feeling of your feet just merging into the floor. Feel this white, puffy cloud of light, this relaxing sense of calm, feel it now as it moves up into your legs. Let it move gradually along your shins and feel it as it softly massages and kneads the muscles there in your calves. Feel your legs becoming very limp and loose now, as all the tension drains from them. Let go in your knee joints and in your thighs. As you let go in your thighs, just imagine this billowy cloud of light moving through your thighs, lulling all your muscles there to relax; softening them into a state of peace and calm. As you let go in your thighs, you might notice that your thighs begin to part a bit, and that's okay. Just imagine all the tension of the day, all concerns you may have, just feel all of this being drained away through your thighs and channeled out from your body. Focus now on your buttocks and, as you inhale, I want you to squeeze the muscles there in your buttocks—squeeze them tightly. Squeeze the muscles in your buttocks and your abdomen and pelvic area. Squeeze tightly now. As you exhale, release and gently let go. Just let it all hang loose and feel that wonderful sense of peace that comes as you release the tightness and allow the softness, the peace, the stillness to set in. Feel the sense of peace and comfort now in your abdominal area; that area that can hang onto so much tightness and so much tension. Feel the muscles in your abdomen now just soften and loosen and let go. Just imagine all the little organs there in your abdomen breathing a collective sigh of relief as all the tension just drains away now and they are left afloat in a sea of peaceful calm. Know that as you deepen into this state of serenity and peace, that all fear just dissipates; for fear and peace cannot coexist. As you relax, as you become still, you are at peace. Feel this white, puffy cloud of light, this relaxing sense of calm, feel it now, as it moves up into your chest area and, as you inhale now, just imagine you are drawing this beautiful cloud of light into your lungs. And, as you exhale, just let your entire rib cage softly fall, softly fall into this beautiful cloud of light. Notice now, how much smoother, how much gentler your breathing is now. As you focus on your breathing once more, notice the peace and the tranquility that there is now, as you breathe in and breathe out, breathe in and breathe out, breathe in and breathe out. Imagine this white, puffy cloud of light, this relaxing sense of calm, imagine it now flowing along your breast bone, feel it as it moves up into your shoulders now, soothing and smoothing away whatever pockets of tension might be stored there. And, as you relax in your shoulders, you might notice that your shoulders begin to droop a bit, and that's okay. Hold onto nothing. Hold onto nothing except this wonderful sense of relaxation and peace that you are experiencing now. Allow this relaxing sense of calm now to spill over into your upper back, that area that can hang onto so much tension and so much tightness. Feel the muscles there in your upper back now just give way to this sense of peace and feel all the tightness there begin to unfurl. Let all the tension just fade away. Imagine this beautiful cloud of light, this wonderful sense of calm, imagine it now, cascading all the way down your spinal column; and, as you release in your spine, just imagine that your vertebrae, one by one, begin to sink deeper and deeper and deeper into the calm. Now prepare for the last vestiges of tension to be removed from your upper body, as you focus now on your arms, and imagine this white, puffy cloud of light, imagine it now, as it floats down your upper arms, feel it as it flows into your elbows, down now into your forearms. Let it stream now into your wrists and flow ever so gently now into the palms of your hands, all the way out the very tips of your fingers. Just feel your arms becoming so heavy now, as all the tension just fades away. You might notice now that your shoulders may even droop more now as you find it harder and harder to resist the pull to let go and relax. You might even notice that the tips of your fingers begin to tingle a bit, as the last vestiges of tension drain through them.

You are doing so well now. Your body is responding so perfectly. Continue now, in this state, letting nothing distract you. Close the door on any unwanted thoughts. And any outside noises that you might hear will only serve to move you further and further away and deeper and deeper into this state of stillness and peace.

Feel this white, puffy cloud of light, this relaxing sense of calm, feel it now, as it moves up into your neck area, and allow the muscles there at the base of your head just to loosen and let go. You might notice that this causes your head to tilt forward a bit, and that's okay. Just let go. Feel this sense of stillness now, as it comes over your throat area. And just imagine your vocal cords at rest now, all movement around your throat stilled—silenced by this beautiful sense of calm. Let go in your jaw and, as you let go in your jaw, your lips might part a bit and that's okay. Again, hold onto nothing. Feel this wonderful sense of peace now, as it permeates your mouth. Feel the quietness and the stillness settling in at the back of your throat. Notice how comfortable it is to have your tongue resting so quietly on the floor of your mouth or nestled against your upper palate. Feel this relaxing sense of calm, this white, puffy cloud of light, as it moves upward now into your face. Feel it as it begins to pulsate along your cheekbones, spanning out now, to touch that area around your temples and your ears. Imagine that you can feel yourself being gently massaged around your temples, encouraged to just let go. Feel all the tension draining now from your face, all traces of tightness or tautness just fading away. Feel this relaxing sense of calm, this white, puffy cloud of light, feel it now as it begins to move along the bridge of your nose, feel it as it streams out now to touch the areas there around your eyes, and feel the muscles there, in the corners of your eyes, just loosen and let go and free themselves of any tightness you might have been carrying there. Relax the area in between your brow. As you loosen and free yourself of all traces of tension in your face, you might notice that your face becomes a bit warm, much as if you had your face turned to the rays of the sun and it was beaming softly down upon you. Feel this sense of calm now as it moves up into your forehead, soothing and smoothing away whatever tightness or tension you might be carrying there. Let this sensation comfort you, much as if a gentle hand was softly stroking your brow. And finally, allow this relaxing sense of calm, this white, puffy cloud of light, allow it now to move up into your scalp area, smoothing away whatever tightness or tension you might be carrying on the surface of your head. In your mind's eye now, just imagine this white, puffy cloud of light, imagine it seeping down into the very pores of your scalp. Allow it to infiltrate the innermost recesses of your mind, sweeping away whatever tension-filled thoughts or fear-filled emotions that might be stored there. And, as this beautiful sense of relaxation and calm flows unencumbered now, just imagine your entire mind being bathed in clarity and light and filled with images and thoughts of comfort, serenity, and peace.

You are so relaxed now, from the top of your head, to the very tips of your toes, you are at peace. Calm in mind, calm in heart, calm in body.

Visualization Script

You are so relaxed. Your whole being is so tranquil and still. It's as if someone has turned out all the lights in the house you call your body, and all your muscles, cells, and organs are fast asleep, nestled into a state of calm repose and rest. No matter what may be occurring on the outside, hold this image of your body being totally relaxed and at peace. Pay close attention to your breathing. Breathe slowly, in and out, through your nose. Breathe evenly, slowly, gently. Let your inhale come softly and then release gently into the exhale, without effort, force, or strain. Let no outer activity distract you; just become lost in the rhythmic flow of your breathing. Notice the feelings and sensations as air flows in and then flows out your body. And now, with each inhale, I want you to imagine that you are being softly swept up; and with each exhale, imagine that you are being gently pushed far, far, away. Feel yourself drifting now, being lifted up and carried away by the movement of your breathing. Inhale, and feel yourself being swept up. Exhale, and let yourself be pushed far, far away.

Now in your mind's eye allow yourself to be transported to a beautiful meadow. It has just rained, and the earth smells of fresh moisture. Breathe deeply and allow the smell of damp earth to penetrate your nostrils. It delights you! You look at the grass and the foliage of the trees and notice that they glisten with newly fallen raindrops—creating the illusion of tiny sunbeams all about you. Everything is so clean, so fresh, so pure. You look down at your feet and notice that nestled there among the glistening blades of grass is a most beautiful rainbow that extends outward from your feet in a small arc, curved like a horseshoe. One end of the rainbow connects with your right foot, and the other end with your left. As you gaze at this rainbow you cannot help but be amazed at how beautiful the colors harmonize and blend with each other. Colors of red, blue, orange, yellow, and green. You can even feel the vibrations of energy emanating from these colors as they softly connect with your feet.

And now let yourself focus on the red ray of the rainbow. It's the color nearest to you. And imagine that as you inhale you are drawing this ray of color in through your feet and up into your body. Feel the flow of the color red as it moves throughout your body like warm liquid light. The color red symbolizes life, strength, power, and vitality. Feel the movement of this color as it travels upward into your body—through your legs and thighs, your hips, your abdomen, your chest, your shoulders. Allow it to move along your back and through your arms. Picture it now as it moves into your neck and face and head. Envelope your body in the color red. Let it pulsate to this color—and as it does, experience your body becoming alive, vital, and strong. And as you feel yourself fully saturated with this red ray of light, let it flow from your body through the crown of your head and form an arch directly above you.

Now focus again on the rainbow at your feet. Inhale deeply and this time draw the color orange into your body. Let it flow into your lower body, upward into your abdomen, into your upper body until you are permeated throughout with the color orange. Orange symbolizes optimism, self-confidence, enthusiasm, and courage. Allow it to flow freely to those areas in your body where you are experiencing doubt or fear. Draw out the courage and optimism you can feel in this color. And now let this color emerge through the top of your head and join the color red in the arch above you.

And now draw in the yellow ray of the rainbow through your feet. Let it rise like warm liquid light and gently flow throughout your being. Yellow symbolizes mental or intellectual power, wisdom, happiness, and joy. Take delight now as you picture your entire body filled with the color yellow. Feel every organ and cell in your body opening to the uplifting, positive, joy-filled vibration of this color. Let this color stream into any areas of your body that are in pain or that ache with sadness. See these areas open like lotus petals to take in the soothing, warm, glowing rays of yellow light. See it infusing every atom, every cell of your body with the wisdom and understanding needed to restore your body to perfect health. And now allow the yellow color to exit your body and join the rays of red and orange arched above your head.

Look down at your feet now and see the green ray of the rainbow preparing to move into your body. Green symbolizes balance, peace, growth, and healing. Allow this color to engulf you, and feel it injecting your entire being with its healing and harmonizing power. As this color flows through your body now, visualize it sparking the growth of new and healthy cells—cells that will quickly outnumber and overpower the confused and unhealthy ones that are causing your illness. Feel harmony and peace being restored in your body and join the trio of colors arched above your head.

You look down at your feet and notice that there is one ray left—the blue. And inhaling now, you pull this beautiful blue ray in through your feet. And as you do so, an even deeper state of tranquility comes over you; a heightened sense of relaxation prevails. Blue symbolizes inspiration, creativity, and faith. Blue calms and cools. Let your body respond to these special qualities of the color blue. Relax. Enjoy the feeling of this soothing, cooling color moving throughout your body. If any part of your body feels inflamed or irritated, envision blue light flowing to that area, cooling, calming, and relaxing. Now let the color blue spiral upward throughout your body and filter out the top of your head to complete the rainbow formed above you.

From the tips of your toes to the top of your head, you have funneled the colors of the rainbow throughout your being, and they have done their healing work. Picture yourself now standing in this beautiful lush meadow with a rainbow of colors crowning your head, with thousands of sunbeams glistening about you, and with the warm moist earth beneath your feet. How special you feel. How special you are! And from deep within you there rises now a sense, an indisputable knowing, that all is well. *All is truly well.*

Inhale deeply now and then softly exhale. Inhale gently and again feel yourself being slowly swept up. Exhale and again experience being drawn away—away this time from the meadow and back into the present awareness. Breathe softly and evenly, taking leave of the meadow, letting the image of you, the image of the rainbow gradually fade. Bring back with you the feeling of specialness, of well-being and peace. Ah yes, those exquisite feelings of well-being and peace and the knowing that all is truly well. Softly, gently, quietly come back. Inhale deeply and feel your eyelids part. Exhale now and fully open your eyes.

To order this tape, please use the form on the last page of this book.

About the Author

Harriett L. Sanders, L.C.S.W., currently serves as Manager of Social Services at the Alta Bates Comprehensive Cancer Center in Berkeley. An experienced practitioner, Harriett conducts relaxation and visualization sessions on an ongoing basis for patients with cancer.

Harriett obtained her B.A. and M.S.W. degrees from Howard University in Washington, D.C. She has worked in the health care field for 24 years—the last 11 of which have been exclusively in oncology.

Other New Harbinger Self-Help Titles

The Warrior's Journey Home: Healing Men, Healing the Planet, $12.95
Weight Loss Through Persistence, $12.95
Post-Traumatic Stress Disorder: A Complete Treatment Guide, $39.95
Stepfamily Realities: How to Overcome Difficulties and Have a Happy Family, $11.95
Leaving the Fold: A Guide for Former Fundamentalists and Others Leaving Their Religion, $12.95
Father-Son Healing: An Adult Son's Guide, $12.95
The Chemotherapy Survival Guide, $11.95
Your Family/Your Self: How to Analyze Your Family System, $11.95
Being a Man: A Guide to the New Masculinity, $12.95
The Deadly Diet, Second Edition: Recovering from Anorexia & Bulimia, $11.95
Last Touch: Preparing for a Parent's Death, $11.95
Consuming Passions: Help for Compulsive Shoppers, $11.95
Self-Esteem, Second Edition, $12.95
Depression & Anxiety Mangement: An audio tape for managing emotional problems, $11.95
I Can't Get Over It, A Handbook for Trauma Survivors, $12.95
Concerned Intervention, When Your Loved One Won't Quit Alcohol or Drugs, $11.95
Redefining Mr. Right, $11.95
Dying of Embarrassment: Help for Social Anxiety and Social Phobia, $11.95
The Depression Workbook: Living With Depression and Manic Depression, $13.95
Risk-Taking for Personal Growth: A Step-by-Step Workbook, $11.95
The Marriage Bed: Renewing Love, Friendship, Trust, and Romance, $11.95
Focal Group Psychotherapy: For Mental Health Professionals, $44.95
Hot Water Therapy: Save Your Back, Neck & Shoulders in 10 Minutes a Day $11.95
Older & Wiser: A Workbook for Coping With Aging, $12.95
Prisoners of Belief: Exposing & Changing Beliefs that Control Your Life, $10.95
Be Sick Well: A Healthy Approach to Chronic Illness, $11.95
Men & Grief: A Guide for Men Surviving the Death of a Loved One., $11.95
When the Bough Breaks: A Helping Guide for Parents of Sexually Abused Childern, $11.95
Love Addiction: A Guide to Emotional Independence, $11.95
When Once Is Not Enough: Help for Obsessive Compulsives, $11.95
The New Three Minute Meditator, $9.95
Getting to Sleep, $10.95
The Relaxation & Stress Reduction Workbook, 3rd Edition, $13.95
Leader's Guide to the Relaxation & Stress Reduction Workbook, $19.95
Beyond Grief: A Guide for Recovering from the Death of a Loved One, $10.95
Thoughts & Feelings: The Art of Cognitive Stress Intervention, $13.95
Messages: The Communication Skills Book, $12.95
The Divorce Book, $11.95
Hypnosis for Change: A Manual of Proven Techniques, 2nd Edition, $12.95
The Chronic Pain Control Workbook, $13.95
Visualization for Change, $12.95
Videotape: Clinical Hypnosis for Stress & Anxiety Reduction, $24.95
My Parent's Keeper: Adult Children of the Emotionally Disturbed, $11.95
When Anger Hurts, $12.95
Free of the Shadows: Recovering from Sexual Violence, $12.95
Lifetime Weight Control, $11.95
The Anxiety & Phobia Workbook, $13.95
Love and Renewal: A Couple's Guide to Commitment, $12.95
The Habit Control Workbook, $12.95

Call **toll free, 1-800-748-6273**, to order. Have your Visa or Mastercard number ready. Or send a check for the titles you want to New Harbinger Publications, Inc., 5674 Shattuck Avenue, Oakland, CA 94609. Include $3.80 for the first book and 75¢ for each additional book, to cover shipping and handling. (California residents please include appropriate sales tax.) Allow four to six weeks for delivery.

Prices subject to change without notice.

Body Relaxed—Mind at Ease

A Relaxing, Calming,
Healing Audio Tape
Combining Peaceful Images
and Serene Music

HARRIETT SANDERS, L.C.S.W.

The Chemotherapy Relaxation Tape

Body Relaxed—Mind at Ease

is a special kind of relaxation tape. The script appearing in Chapter 12 of *The Chemotherapy Survival Guide* was written to help people undergoing chemotherapy to remain calm and peaceful. *Body Relaxed—Mind at Ease* helps you systematically let go of tension in every part of your body. It helps you breathe with a strong, deeply peaceful rhythm. You learn to use images of calming light to replace the hot spots of tension.

The image of the rainbow is used to powerful effect. Each color is identified with a special healing quality: red with strength, orange with courage, yellow with wisdom and joy, green with balance and harmony, blue with calmness. Together these images help to restore a soothing sense of inner peace.

Written by Harriett Sanders, L.C.S.W., this tape is based on years of experience leading hundreds of relaxation groups for people dealing with cancer and chemotherapy. Her voice is a gentle alto that creates confidence and a deep sense of serenity. The tape is backed by the exquisite "Angel Love" by Aeoliah. You'll find that this music beautifully complements Harriett Sanders' healing words.

■ Order Form ■

Complete this form and return it to New Harbinger Publications, Inc., 5674 Shattuck Avenue, Oakland, CA 94609, or phone us at (800) 748-6273, or fax this page to (510) 652-5472.

Please send me _____ copies of *Body Relaxed—Mind at Ease*

Your Name _____

Address _____

City, State, Zip _____

Telephone: Daytime, Mon.-Fri (_____) _____
(In case we need to contact you about your order.)

Check for $11.95 plus $3.80 shipping (Californians add appropriate tax).
Charge to ☐ Visa ☐ Mastercard

Expiration Date_____

Signature _____

Lifetime Guarantee: If not satisfied, return this tape at any time for a full refund, less shipping and handling.